Palliative Care for the Primary Care Team

2

Other titles in the 'Issues for the Palliative Care' series:

Why is it so difficult to die? by Brian Nyatanga

Fundamental Aspects of Palliative Care Nursing by Robert Becker and Richard Gamlin

Hidden Aspects of Palliative Care edited by Brian Nyatanga and Maxine Astley-Pepper

Palliative Care for those with Learning Disabilities edited by Sue Read

Aspects of Social Work and Palliative Care edited by Jonathan Parker

Series editor: Brian Nyatanga

Palliative Care for the Primary Care Team

Eileen Palmer and John Howarth

Quay Books
MA Healthcare Limited

Quay Books Division, MA Healthcare Limited, St Jude's Church, Dulwich Road, London SE24 0PB

British Library Cataloguing-in-Publication Data
A catalogue record is available for this book

Printed in the UK by Ashford Colour Press Limited, Gosport, Hampshire

Contents

Introduction

We only get one chance at it! If we can't cure, we need to do the dying well. We need to reinvent the nineteenth century Victorian model of the good death, and place it back into modern day health and social care structures.

From: *A Good Death — The Last Taboo* by Rabbi Julia Neuberger, presented at the Annual Conference National Forum for Hospice at Home in 2001

This book is designed as a practical handbook for busy GPs and district nurses who may not have had the benefit of training in palliative care.

Ninety per cent of palliative care is done in primary care, and most patients (given the choice) would prefer to die in their own home. The content of this book makes few assumptions about pre-existing knowledge. This reflects the fact that, even as this is written, training in the principles and practice of palliative care at undergraduate or postgraduate level is not a routine or significant part of the nursing or medical curriculum.

Five core themes are repeated throughout this book.

I. The importance and value of the basic therapeutic relationship between patient and health worker

This first theme embodies principles of empathy and respect for the unique individual in front of us who is facing his or her own mortality, in his or her own way. This can sound an impossible goal in a busy week, with multiple complex demands and overstretched resources. However, there are basic, evidence-based skills that can improve the effectiveness and outcome of consultations and, by their nature, help to develop relationships based on genuineness, honesty, integrity, respect and empathy. Primary care has been at the forefront of developing and using these skills in the consultation, and these are the skills that are of most value in the complex merging of medicine and humanity that modern palliative care seeks to provide.

2. The principle of dealing with the patient and support network together

The second theme is the principle of dealing with a patient, not in isolation, but as part of a family and community where the impact of serious illness on any one person will cause effects, ranging from ripples to tidal waves, in the family and social network around that person. Impeccable clinical care for one individual, which ignores the family and social context of that individual, is almost always a disservice. Again, primary care is well placed to contribute a wealth of skill in family medicine.

3. The importance of whole-person care

As doctors and nurses we are taught a great deal about the physical body, something about the mind, a little about the family, and almost nothing about spiritual care. Palliative care seeks to support all of these. The primary care team has a long tradition of multidisciplinary team working. It is pivotal in forming effective referral pathways into secondary care, other community services, and other agencies, such as social services or chaplaincy. The GP can help coordinate the use of these resources, and help the patient to navigate the complex care arrangements. The idea of the GP or community nurse as an advocate for the patient, helping lobby to get the best out of the system, is not new. This advocacy and effective teamworking is seldom more important than in palliative care.

4. Good palliative care is pro-active

The doctor or nurse looks ahead and anticipates. The occupational therapist is brought in before the patient falls. The syringe driver (and the medication needed to go in it) is in the home or easily accessible a day or two before the patient slips into unconsciousness. The family, who otherwise would have been very anxious at this point, are comforted by knowing who to contact and what the plan is. If a difficult pain is anticipated, the local specialist resource is contacted.

5. Good communication is essential

This is so often where things can go so badly wrong. Large multidisciplinary teams spanning primary care, out-of-hours services, secondary care, and social services grow around these patients. Patients and their families also have communication needs. General practices will need robust systems to ensure important information is shared between appropriate team members effectively.

> *Palliative care rarely goes wrong because of a lack of knowledge about subgroups of morphine receptors in the central nervous system; it is usually because of failure in one of these basic five areas. This is the challenge for primary care.*

The palliative care consultation

It is through the consultation that we deliver the majority of care to a patient. A superb organizational framework that facilitates access for the palliative care patient is of little use if the consultation is clumsy or insensitive, and poor care is likely to result.

Consultation skills are taught to current GP registrars. Most, when asked, can recite the different models of the consultation and the contents of a good consultation. Putting it into practice when faced with a dying patient and a family in despair, however, is not so easy. We may have to break bad news, discuss death, explore deep emotions and anger and explain complex management options all in the same consultation. Palliative care consultations can be the most challenging and stretch our skills to the limit. They can also be the most rewarding.

Both the clinician and patient enter consultations with clear agendas and pre-conceived ideas. Most of the time this is useful as it is experience- and knowledge-based, but, occasionally, it can be 'baggage' that gets in the way of an effective consultation. We may well not be able to change our own baggage, or that of the patient, but we can try to understand it, find a way round it and make sure that it does not get in the way of good care.

The palliative care consultation may enter areas where the clinician feels far from comfortable. The emotional pain felt by the patient and his or her carers is sometimes palpable; however professional we are, we cannot avoid being affected. We often mirror the patient's own feelings. It is useful to reflect back on a consultation and ask, 'How did that make me feel?' If we left feeling anxious, powerless and depressed, we are often feeling the same things as the patient. This can be emotionally draining and we can end up feeling that the situation is hopeless and nothing can be done. We will also reflect this emotion back on the patient, making them feel even more helpless and frightened.

A theme repeated in this book is that there is always something that can be done. We should be positive about what can be done, and we should not remove hope. Hope is an important coping tool. It is quite possible for a patient to understand intellectually that the situation is terminal but, at the same time emotionally, to continue to hope that things will get better. Some clinicians see it as their role to force reality on a patient, to make them acknowledge that the situation is terminal, to remove hope because it is not realistic. We advocate a gentler approach that is more patient-led. Patients' apparent lack of realism about the situation may be their way of coping with it, and their acceptance of the terminal nature of the illness may be gradual.

It is also important not to forget the therapeutic importance of the consultation itself; 'I felt so much better after we last discussed it'. By remaining positive, constructive, practical and being credible and professional, we reflect these emotions back to the patient, rather than emotions of uncertainty and hopelessness. Remaining positive is also important for our own personal survival; if we left every consultation feeling despair, we would not last long in the job.

> *What is dying like? Well, there are no more health worries, no more career worries and you can forget pension plans. Of course, that's both liberating and isolating. I suppose you don't quite belong anymore. Its marked by the fact that some friends run a million miles, but also by countless acts of kindness. The cup is always half full. Death has no power over memory. It has no power over love. Death has no dominion. Nothing can be taken away from us.*
>
> Patient with anaplastic carcinoma of the maxillary antrum

The normal working day of most primary care workers is sadly dominated by time pressure. We have to be careful when we take this time management agenda into the palliative care consultation. Having one eye on the clock and looking for opportunities to close a consultation has become a necessary feature at times in general practice, especially when dealing with minor illness. Saving time with some consultations frees up time for others, and should not be seen as a bad thing, unless it begins to dominate every consultation.

However, when dealing with palliative care we need to change our mindset. We cannot let the time management agenda dominate, and have to organize access for these patients in a different way. A five-minute consultation in the middle of an emergency surgery is seldom conducive to good palliative care. Double or longer appointments may be necessary at the end of a surgery when there are fewer time constraints. A home visit may be needed and will give insight into the home and family situation that may be missed when the patient is seen out of context in the surgery. It is not possible to deal with every issue at every consultation. A 'rolling' consultation over weeks and months with multiple contacts is needed, picking up from where we left off and adapting to the changing situation. Consultations can take place in the surgery, during a home visit, by telephone or even by e-mail. Often a combination of these is highly effective, the balance between them changing as the patient deteriorates.

Most clinicians start a consultation with an open question, such as 'how are you?', and then listen carefully. It is particularly important not to close the consultation down too quickly, and several open questions may be needed, such as 'how are you coping?' or 'how are the family managing?' It is easy to focus too quickly on the physical symptoms and miss the fact that the patient is depressed or the family is in crisis.

As the consultation progresses we form various hypotheses and test them out by asking specific closed questions, such as 'is the pain worse if you breathe deeply?' Doctors are trained to make a diagnosis. What we are doing, however, is based on probabilities, and we live with varying degrees of uncertainty. In a dying patient, when extensive investigation may not be appropriate, the degree of uncertainty increases and we often end up treating a symptom rather than a confirmed diagnosis. In palliative care, we need to be constantly reassessing and challenging our hypotheses; for example, vomiting may be caused by constipation initially but, as the disease progresses, hypercalcaemia may begin to contribute.

The consultation is not a linear process — it ebbs and flows. Several hypotheses may be chased up with closed questioning punctuated by mini-summaries and further open questions, such as 'how do you feel in yourself?' It is like a conversation, and the skilled clinician knows when to keep quiet and listen, when to prompt, when to pick up on cues, when to summarize and when to draw it to a close. Being patient-centred does not mean that the consultation should just drift, it still needs some structure. If difficult issues are raised or emotions triggered, we should not just leave things up in the air: there needs to be a clear end to the consultation, with a summary and positive plan of action.

A review should be arranged; do not just leave it for the patient to ring back if needed. A palliative situation needs regular review to be pro-active and anticipate the next step, rather than simply reactive to crises. This review can be shared between members of the primary care team. Safety netting is of particular importance in the palliative care setting. Most safety netting is too vague, for example, 'ring me if you need me', and does not help the patient make a decision on when to get help. Be specific: 'I plan to review you next week, but in the meantime you should be calling us if this, this or this happens'. There is little point in good safety netting if the patient rings and cannot get an appointment. Access for this group of patients should be facilitated, for example, by a rapid access prompt on their notes or special patient details sent to the 'out-of-hours' provider.

The consultation should be documented clearly, though we still have the situation where different primary care workers use different sets of notes. Communication between team members is discussed further in *Chapter 24* on the organization of care.

While the consultation needs to be patient-centred, it does not need to be entirely patient-led. There are certain common problems that need to be actively searched for, and their presence or absence clearly documented.

Dr Eileen Palmer and Dr John Howarth
January, 2005

Acknowledgements

The authors appreciate and would like to acknowledge the support and encouragement we have received from our families, friends and professional colleagues.

Special thanks are due to:

~ West Cumbria Hospice at Home
~ North Cumbria Syringe Driver Protocol Steering Group
~ Dr Tim Sowton, Macmillan GP facilitator, North Cumbria
~ Margaret Ross, Community Macmillan Nurse, North Cumbria
~ Bernice O'Connor, Hospice at Home nurse, West Cumbria Hospice at Home
~ Ros Dickinson, Hospice at Home nurse, West Cumbria Hospice at Home
~ Jean Radley, Anglican priest
~ Fred Lightfoot
~ Mary Dixon
~ Marion Stevenson-Rouse
~ Each and every one of our patients, who are our real inspiration, and to whom this book is dedicated.

Part 1
Physical

1

The principles of symptom control in palliative care

There are certain core principles in managing all symptoms in palliative care.

Assess the whole patient

- How ill are they?
- What is their likely life expectancy?
- Where are they on the journey?
- How interventionist do they wish their treatment to be?
- What is their preferred care setting?
- What are their priorities, including emotional and spiritual issues?
- What is the view of the family?
- How can we use our limited resources effectively?

Correct the correctable

- It is important to recognize that many symptoms can be corrected
- Not all symptoms are caused by the cancer
- Do not let the situation run out of control; try to anticipate. Think ahead, plan the next step and get timely help and advice.

Manage the incorrectable

- Incorrectable problems engender a feeling of helplessness for patients, families and the caring professionals
- Even apparently hopeless situations can be managed; there is always something that can be done to manage the problem. This is an important point in the whole approach to apparently hopeless situations
- Patients and families value compassion and support enormously
- A starting point is a careful, honest explanation of the symptoms and their possible causes
- Always balance difficult information with positive, constructive comments.... 'This is what is happening *but* we can do this, this and this to help you feel better'.

2

Pain

Pain is not inevitable in cancer

About one-quarter of patients with cancer never have pain. Of those who do, one-third have a single pain, and another third have three or more different pains. Eighty percent of cancer pain can be controlled using oral analgesics (see *Chapter 2.2* Using the World Health Organization [WHO] analgesic ladder, *p. 10*), yet many patients with cancer continue to experience unnecessary pain.

Primary healthcare teams are ideally placed to ensure all their patients with cancer have access to satisfactory pain control. The route to satisfactory pain control involves:

- asking every patient about pain
- hearing the response
- knowing the common causes of pain in cancer
- understanding that pain in cancer is often complicated by fear of its meaning; both need to be addressed for good pain control
- using a strong opioid in a skilled way at the right time
- using co-analgesics appropriately
- ensuring continuity and follow up
- knowing when to ask for help and where to get it.

There is evidence that:

- health workers, such as doctors and nurses, tend to underestimate pain
- families tend to overestimate pain.

> The patient is the most accurate judge of the pain experienced:
>
> 'Pain is what the patient says it is'.

We have to be realistic and set goals that are achievable:

- **pain relief at night should always be achievable**
- **pain relief during the day should usually be achieveable**
- **pain relief with activity is not always possible, but should be striven for.**

2.1 Pain assessment

Assessment of pain is the first step. Assessment is vital to work out the likely cause of the pain; this then defines the best management strategy. Diagnose the pain before you treat; it may need more than just simple analgesia.

Real life examples

⌘ Pain from an impending pathological fracture in a previously independent woman with metastatic breast cancer needed urgent referral for orthopaedic stabilization and radiotherapy, following which she was pain-free on a small dose of morphine.

⌘ A rapidly escalating pain in a middle-aged man with newly diagnosed lung cancer responded poorly to a rapid escalation in his morphine dose. The GP sat down and talked through the implications of his diagnosis and his fears and concerns with him and his wife. His pain settled completely and his morphine dose was reduced.

Pain in cancer may be caused by:

- the cancer itself
- cancer treatments
- immobility/weakness
- something totally unrelated to cancer.

The latter is often overlooked by both doctor and patient, who may assume all pain represents disease progression. Pain is a complex experience with physical, psychological, social and spiritual components. Accurate assessment looks at the whole patient (*Table 2.1.1*).

Table 2.1.1: Whole-patient pain assessment	
Physical	What is the likely cause of this pain in this patient at this time? What structural or functional abnormality would cause this pain pattern?
Psychological	How is the patient coping with the pain? How much anxiety or depression is present? What are the patient's ideas, concerns or expectations about pain and its management in this situation? What information do they need?
Social	How is the pain affecting the family? How much family anxiety is present? What are the family's ideas, concerns and expectations? (These may differ from the patient's) How have family dynamics been affected by this illness? How is the pain limiting the usual role(s)?
Spiritual	How much distress or suffering is this patient experiencing? What does the pain mean to them? What does the illness mean to them? What sustains them in difficult times?

Taking a pain history

Accurate pain assessment starts by taking a good history:

1. Ask the patient 'Where is your pain?'; 'Show me where you feel the pain'; 'How long have you had the pain?'
2. Record the site, duration and intensity of each pain
3. What has already been tried by patient and clinician, and with what effect?

Site of pain

Using a simple body chart to document the location and intensity of pain(s) at first assessment can form a useful *aide memoir* and be valuable in monitoring the effectiveness of interventions, particularly when dealing with multiple pains (see *Figure 2.1.1*).

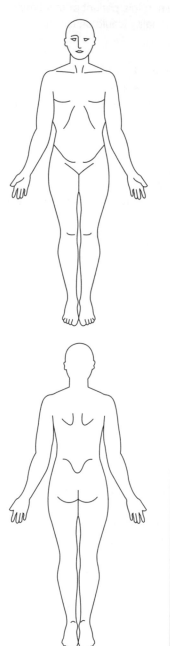

Pain	Symptoms	1 2 3 4
Intensity	Mild	
	Moderate	
	Severe	
	Overwhelming	
Duration	1–2 weeks	
	2–6 weeks	
	6–12 weeks	
	>12 weeks	
Periodicity	Constant	
	Intermittent	
Effect on	Sleep	
	Mobility	
Effect of present medication	No difference	
	Partial control	
	Complete control	
Other treatment	Nerve block	
	Radiotherapy	
	Other	
Effect	No difference	
	Partial control	
	Complete control	

Relatives' views:

Other information:

Possible causes of each pain:

1

2

3

4

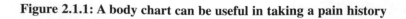

Figure 2.1.1: A body chart can be useful in taking a pain history

Duration of pain

The duration of pain should be recorded: 'Is it episodic or continuous?'; 'Was there a clear trigger, eg. a fall or a certain movement?' (see *Figure 2.1.1*).

Intensity of pain

A simple measure of pain intensity is to ask the patient 'What does the pain stop you doing?', and 'Does the pain disturb your sleep?' Various pain-intensity scales are available and can be useful where staff and patients are well trained. These grade pain intensity on numerical or verbal visual analogue scales (see *Figure 2.1.1*).

Do not forget that pain does not just have physical components. The doctor or nurse should be alert to emotional cues from the patient or family in their appearance, behaviour or choice of words. Does the patient appear angry or frightened? Is he or she tired, withdrawn or depressed? Is he or she expressing negative thoughts or hopelessness? The doctor or nurse should also record relatives' views and any other information relevant to the patient.

Recognising common pain patterns

There are some common pain patterns that are worth learning to recognize and differentiate clinically:

- visceral pain
- bone pain
- nerve pain
- colic
- cutaneous pain.

Recognising these common pain patterns enables the appropriate use of strong opioids and also co-analgesics. It enables the early identification of situations where other treatment modalities, such as radiotherapy, have a major role. It also allows explanation to patient and family, and establishes confidence that the symptom is being addressed skilfully and professionally. This is an important first step in engaging patient and family in a jointly agreed management plan.

Visceral pain

This is poorly localized, diffuse and often aching in quality.

Bone pain

This is well localized, and there may be localized bony tenderness. Movement and weight-bearing classically exacerbate bone pain. If this feature is pronounced it may suggest impending pathological fracture, and the affected area should be rested until an X-ray can be arranged. Bone pain has a high index of suspicion with cancers that commonly metastasize to bone (cancers of the breast, bronchus, prostate, kidney and myeloma).

Nerve pain

This follows a dermatonal distribution. Nerve pain is pathognomic. It is often described as burning, tingling, jabbing or stabbing, and may be associated with disordered sensation or motor weakness. Patients find nerve pain unpleasant. It can be difficult to manage with the usual painkillers, and early liaison with a specialist palliative care or pain team is recommended.

Colic

Colic comes and goes in spasms, which last from seconds to minutes. Bowel colic is often described as windy or griping pain by patients. It is poorly relieved by opioids, but well relieved by anti-spasmodics.

Cutaneous pain

This is a well-localized superficial pain. The commonest aetiology is pressure damage to skin.

Managing some common pain patterns

The first step is always to follow the WHO analgesic ladder (see *Section 2.2, p. 12*), rapidly using a strong opioid if necessary. However, in bone pain, nerve pain, colic and cutaneous pain, additional interventions are almost always necessary. Do not delay initiating these additional measures (such as radiotherapy for bone pain). Again, it comes back to the importance of a clear diagnosis of the pain, and good anticipatory care.

Table 2.1.2 outlines the different interventions for each of the five common pain patterns outlined above.

Table 2.1.2: Interventions for the five common pain patterns

Pain pattern	Morphine responsiveness	Useful co-analgesics	Other interventions
Visceral pain	Usually completely responsive*	Not usually required	Not usually required
Bone pain	Often good response	NSAIDs (sometimes steroids)	Radiotherapy Bisphosphonate infusions Surgical stabilization
Nerve pain	Partial response	Steroids Tricyclic antidepressants Anticonvulsants	Sometimes radiotherapy Early referral for specialist advice
Colic	Partial response	Hyoscine butylbromide (Buscopan™)	(Rarely) surgical relief of obstruction
Cutaneous pain	Often little response (case reports of topical use being helpful)	NSAIDS Topical local anaesthetics	Radiotherapy Eradicating infection Appropriate dressings For pressure sores prevention is better than cure

*Pancreatic pain is the exception, probably because of early involvement of retroperitoneal tissue. As well as morphine, try non-steroidal anti-inflammatory drugs (NSAIDs) and steroids (see text below), and consider early referral to a pain anaesthetic service for coeliac plexus or splanchnic nerve block

Key points

❖ Pain is not inevitable in cancer.

❖ Eighty percent of cancer pain can be managed with oral analgesics using the WHO analgesic ladder (see *Section 2.2*, below).

❖ Primary healthcare teams are ideally placed to set up systems to ensure all their cancer patients have access to satisfactory pain control.

❖ Pain is a complex experience with physical, psychological, social and spiritual components. Accurate assessment looks at the whole patient.

❖ The patient is the most accurate judge of the pain experienced: 'Pain is what the patient says it is'.

❖ Recognizing common pain patterns helps pain management to be better planned.

2.2 Using the WHO analgesic ladder

The WHO analgesic ladder is a simple and well-established tool to determine when to start a strong opioid for cancer pain (see *Figure 2.2.1*).

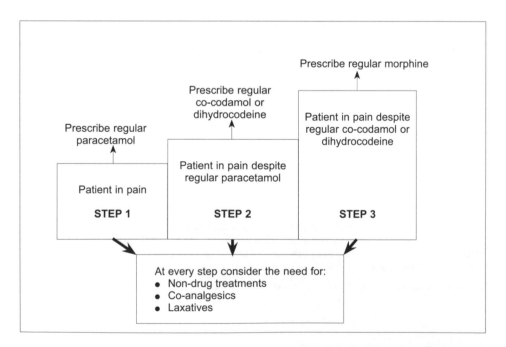

Figure 2.2.1: The WHO analgesic ladder. By using the WHO analgesic ladder, 80–90% of cancer pain will be controlled

The WHO analgesic ladder is simple, and starts with regular paracetamol. If this does not work, use a regular dose of a weak opioid such as co-dydramol, dihydrocodeine, co-codamol or tramadol. If this fails to work, prescribe morphine. There is good evidence that this is both safe and effective.

In practice many patients with cancer pain get 'stuck'; maybe switch from one weak opioid to another several times over a matter of weeks or even months in the attempt to delay 'starting morphine'. During this time, pain control can be unsatisfactory, leading to frustration and loss of confidence.

Understanding the reasons for delaying the introduction of morphine are important.

Patient's concerns about starting morphine

⌘   Fears it will lose its effectiveness 'later on when I really need it'.
⌘   Worries about addiction.
⌘   Thinks morphine will make him or her too sleepy.
⌘   Thinks he or she may be unable to drive or enjoy a drink.
⌘   Thinks it means he or she has not long to live.
⌘   Big transition. Clear daily external confirmation of seriousness of illness
    — a big step on the inner cancer journey.

Doctor's concerns about prescribing morphine

⌘   May share these fears about addiction and tolerance.
⌘   May feel it is 'not the right time' to discuss the use of morphine in case
    the patient 'takes it the wrong way'.
⌘   May worry about side-effects.
⌘   Feels the patient is 'not ill enough'.
⌘   May be sensitive to where the patient is in his or her illness journey and
    choose to pace the step, as in breaking bad news.

Few other medicines carry such complex psychological baggage with them! Pain in cancer is complicated by the fear of its meaning. Prescribing for pain in cancer is complicated by the fears that surround the use of morphine.

> Morphine is nothing more and nothing less than a strong painkiller. It is a naturally occurring product. Used correctly it can neither shorten nor lengthen your life. It has a very good chance of taking your pain away and improving the quality of your life.

Myths about morphine

1. Myth: morphine is addictive
Fact: addiction is rare when treating cancer pain with opioids.
A retrospective review demonstrated that of 24,000 patients with no history of addiction who received opioids for cancer pain, only seven became addicted (Friedman, 1990).
Fact: cancer patients can stop taking opioids when the pain stops (American Pain Society, 1992).
Fact: WHO states 'the medical use of opioids is rarely associated with psychological dependence' (WHO, 1990).

2. Myth: opioids are dangerous
Fact: the safety of opioids in long-term use is well documented. The most prevalent serious side effect is constipation. Chronic use of non-opioids can cause stomach, kidney and liver damage.

There is good evidence for the safety and efficacy of morphine in the control of cancer pain.
There is no evidence that its use in appropriate doses alters life expectancy, nor does it cause clinically significant respiratory depression when used to control pain (Portenoy, 1995).

Before prescribing morphine it is important to encourage the patient and family to voice their fears and concerns and to discuss them in an open and honest manner. What may seem a simple step for health professionals, represents another big and confirming step for patients on their inner journey of trying to come to terms with what is happening. Sometimes this sort of step needs pacing; it may help to give a warning shot.

For example, when one GP starts patients on an intermediate (step 2) analgesic or non-steroidal anti-inflammatory drug (NSAID), he always says 'we will see how you get on with these, but sometimes pain can be better managed with a small dose of a strong painkiller like morphine rather than a big dose of a weaker one'. The patient is prepared for the next step and internally can start to move on. This is similar to the overall approach to breaking bad news.

It may be helpful to sit down as a practice team and discuss each team member's own attitudes to the use of strong opioids, so patients receive a consistent and confident message. A lot of good work can easily be undone by a careless throwaway remark by a team member with doubts, despite the evidence.

Additional written information answering common concerns for patients and professionals is useful. An example is included *pp. 21–23.*

Real life example

Mr F had pelvic recurrence of bowel cancer and was complaining of a dull, constant pain in the lower abdomen. He had self-medicated with his wife's paracetamol, which had given incomplete relief. One of the partners had prescribed some regular dihydrocodeine, which had been a bit better than the paracetamol, but had left him constipated and still in pain. The doctor in the surgical outpatient department had suggested trying co-codamol instead.

Mr F made another appointment, worried that his pain was no better. He thought this lack of improvement and the constipation meant his cancer was much worse. His usual GP was able to explain to him that co-codamol was no stronger than the dihydrocodeine, and that both could cause constipation.

After discussion, Mr F was started on a modified-release morphine formulation (30 mg every twelve hours) along with softener/stimulant laxatives, and was pain-free within twenty-four hours, with control of his constipation a day later.

2.3 Morphine formulations: immediate-release and modified-release

Oral morphine formulations are divided into:

- immediate-release (IR) formulations, which peak within twenty to thirty minutes of oral administration and last about four hours
- modified-release (MR) formulations, which take about four hours to peak and last about twelve hours (or twenty-four hours in the case of MXL) (*Table 2.3.1*).

2.4 Prescribing morphine

Morphine is prescribed by starting with a small, regular dose, which is increased in 30–50% increments until the patient is either pain-free or until further increments are prevented by unacceptable side-effects.

The dose continues to be titrated up according to the clinical response:

there is no dosage ceiling apart from the patient's ability to tolerate the drug.

In primary care, treatment is often initiated with MR morphine, which is more convenient for patient and family. This can work well provided care is taken to ensure that adequate IR morphine is available, and that the patient and family are instructed to use it as necessary during the dose stabilization period.

Occasionally, it is better to start with IR morphine if:

- there is a lot of concern about starting morphine
- the patient is elderly or frail
- the pain is severe.

If there are unacceptable side-effects, at least the dose will wear off after four hours. It is also possible to titrate the dose up much more quickly and responsively.

Both methods are given below.

Table 2.3.1: Morphine formulations: immediate release and modified release

Type	Immediate-release (IR)	Modified-release (MR)	Modified-release (MR) (24-hour)
Duration	4 hours (3–6 hours)	12 hours	24 hours
Time to onset	20–30 minutes (15–60 minutes)	4 hours (1–6 hours)	
Examples	• Morphine oral solution Can be made to any strength	• MST Continus tablets (5 mg, 10 mg, 15 mg, 30 mg, 60 mg, 100 mg,	• Morphgesic SR tablets (10 mg, 30 mg, 60 mg, 100 mg)
	• Oramorph oral solution (10 mg/5 ml)	200 mg) • MST Continus suspension	• Morcap SR capsules (20 mg, 50 mg 100 mg)
	• Oramorph unit dose vials (10 mg, 30 mg, 100 mg)	(20 mg, 30 mg, 60 mg, 100 mg, 200 mg)	• MXL capsules (30 mg, 60 mg, 90 mg, 120 mg,
	• Oramorph concentrated solution (100 mg/5 ml with dropper)	• Zomorph capsules (10 mg, 30 mg, 60 mg, 100 mg, 200 mg)	150 mg)
	• Sevredol tablets (10 mg, 20 mg, 50 mg)		
Used for	Initial dose titration	Continuous pain relief	Continuous pain relief
	Breakthrough pain		
	Incident pain		

Starting morphine (*Table 2.3.2*)

Table 2.3.2.: Regimen used for commencing morphine		
Starting with	**12-hourly modified-(MR) morphine**	**4-hourly immediate-release (IR) morphine**
Starting dose	10–30 mg MR morphine every 12 hours	5–10 mg IR morphine every 4 hours
Additional starting dose as required	5–10 mg IR morphine	5–10 mg IR morphine
Typical increments	20–30–40–60–90–130–160–200 mg every 12 hours, etc	15–20–30–40–60–80–100–120–160–200 mg every 4 hours, etc
Interval between increments	2–3 days	24 hours
Once pain control stable	Maintain on 12-hour MR morphine Monitor at least weekly	Convert to 12-hour MR morphine (total daily dose in mg divided by 2) Check/adjust if necessary after 24 hours

In addition to *Table 2.3.2*, always remember 'ABC' *(Figure 2.3.1)*.

A nti-emetic. *Always* prescribe prophylactically to prevent the morphine-induced nausea and vomiting that can affect one-third of patients in the first seven to ten days of treatment. Haloperidol 1.5–3 mg daily as a single dose is suitable.

B reakthrough pain. *Always* prescribe IR morphine as 'rescue' medication. Use one-sixth of the total twenty-four-hour dose of morphine in mg to use as required (up to hourly).

C onstipation. *Always* prescribe a stimulant and a softener laxative.

Figure 2.3.1: Always remember 'ABC'

Converting to twelve-hourly morphine is easy; add up the twenty-four-hour dose in mg and divide by two. Similarly, to convert to once-daily morphine, add up the twenty-four-hour dose of morphine in mg. Convenient dosing schedules for patients will fit in with bedtime/breakfast, for example 10am/10pm or 9am/9pm.

MR preparations are **not** designed for more frequent dosing. If there is end-of-dose pain, the dose usually needs increasing and the dosage frequency should be left unchanged. (Rarely, some patients appear to be fast metabolizers of morphine and need more frequent dosing, but this is the exception rather than the rule.)

Most patients can expect to be pain-free on a regular, twelve-hourly dose of oral MR morphine. Some patients will also need co-analgesics or non-drug interventions. A small proportion of patients will have difficult pain, which may need multiple specialist interventions and may not be possible to control completely.

Managing severe pain (rapid dose escalation method)

- ⌘ Prescribe IR morphine 5–10 mg every four hours, and 5–10 mg as required.
- ⌘ Encourage to use extra 5–10 mg dose as necessary, making a note of response and level of drowsiness.
- ⌘ Make telephone contact or revisit within first few hours to check response.
- ⌘ Every twenty-four hours calculate the total morphine dose in mg over that twenty-four hours and divide by six. This gives the next incremental dose, which again is prescribed four-hourly and as required.
- ⌘ This process can be repeated every twenty-four hours until the patient is pain-free or too drowsy to tolerate further dose increases.
- ⌘ Once pain control is stable, convert to a long-acting preparation.

Advantages of rapid dose escalation method

- ⌘ Rapid dose escalation, so quicker pain control.
- ⌘ Patient controls rate of dose escalation *vs* side-effects.
- ⌘ Encourages daily assessment by doctor or nurse (can be by telephone for some patients), building confidence and pre-empting problems.
- ⌘ If dose is higher than the patient needs, its effect will wear off in four hours.
- ⌘ Once stable dose requirement established, patient can be accurately transferred onto twelve-hourly morphine or comparable dose of alternative strong opioid with predictable pain control.

Disadvantages of rapid dose escalation method

⌘ Can be confusing for patient unless clear instruction given.
⌘ Needs daily assessment — can put pressure on the team for a few days.
⌘ Needs clear communication between team members.
⌘ Requires patient/carer documentation to be accurate.

Example

John had excruciating right-sided chest pain from a carcinoma of the lung. He had not called the GP, but had self-medicated with paracetamol and a proprietary non-steroidal anti-inflammatory drug; 'I didn't want to be a nuisance, doctor'. He wants to be managed at home, if possible. Dr F prescribed IR morphine 5 mg four-hourly and 5 mg as required, telling John and his wife to:

• take a dose every four hours, whether the pain is there or not
• take an extra dose at any time in between if the pain is still severe
• to make a note of the time and quantity of each dose
• to note its effect after half an hour or so
• to double the dose after two doses if it is having little or no effect
• to phone for advice if he feels too sleepy or is worried what to do.

Dr F leaves these instructions written in the house with a contact number for himself and the nurse. He also prescribes haloperidol and an appropriate laxative, and arranges to telephone in four hours' time. When he telephones, things are a little easier. John had slight ease from the first dose of morphine. He took 5 mg more an hour later, and another 5 mg an hour after that. He is not drowsy and has no side effects, but he is still in pain.

Dr F suggests the dose is doubled to 10 mg, which John and his wife had wondered about doing. He reminds them about the laxatives and to telephone if either of them feels John is becoming too sleepy. The nurse visits the next day. John has continued to need 10 mg doses of morphine every four hours and has also had five 'extra' 10 mg doses.

Over the first twenty-four hours John has had:

• three lots of 5 mg doses
• ten lots of 10 mg doses.

This is 115 mg of IR morphine over twenty-four hours. He is much more comfortable, but not yet pain-free. He is not excessively sleepy. The nurse divides this twenty-four-hour dose by six, which she calculates to be just under 20 mg IR morphine. She suggests that over the next twenty-four hours, John takes 20 mg IR morphine four-hourly with additional doses as necessary, again telephoning for advice if concerned.

John and his wife do not telephone. When the GP revisits the following day, John is pain-free. He has used:

- six lots of 20 mg regular doses
- three lots of 20 mg extra doses.

This is 180 mg over twenty-four hours.

Dr F divides this by six, giving 30 mg every four hours. He suggests this new dose. Once John is stable on it for twenty-four hours he is converted to twelve-hourly MR morphine. (His total daily dose is 180 mg every twenty-four hours. Dividing this by two gives 90 mg of MR morphine every twelve hours.)

Key points

- ❖ The WHO analgesic ladder is a simple and well-established tool to determine when to start a strong opioid for cancer pain.
- ❖ In practice, few other medicines carry such complex psychological baggage as morphine for both doctor and patient.
- ❖ Starting morphine is a big step for patients and their inner perception of their illness.
- ❖ Morphine is prescribed by starting with a small, regular dose, which is increased in 30–50% increments until the patient is either pain free or further increments are prevented by unacceptable side effects.
- ❖ The dose continues to be titrated up according to the clinical response; there is no dosage ceiling apart from the patient's ability to tolerate the drug.
- ❖ A key skill is familiarity with an IR and MR morphine formulation and their correct uses and prescribing.
- ❖ All patients on morphine or strong opioids should routinely be prescribed an anti-emetic and a laxative.

Checklist for the prescription of morphine for chronic pain

1. **Have I prescribed the right dose?**
   There is no 'standard' dose of oral morphine. The dose ranges from
   2.5mg four-hourly to 50mg four-hourly (sometimes more). Most patients
   need less than 30mg four-hourly. The oral route should be used wherever
   possible.

   Start with 5–10mg morphine four-hourly and increase every twenty-four hours
   until the pain is **at least** 90% controlled.

   Typical dose increments: 10>15>20>30>40>60>80>100>120>160>200 MG

2. **Have I prescribed a regular, four-hourly dose?**

3. **Have I remembered A-B-C?** Anti-emetic
   Breakthrough pain, and
   Constipation

   **Have I prescribed 50–100% of the regular four-hourly dose to be
   used prn for breakthrough pain?**

   Have I prescribed a laxative?
   (Co-danthramer or Co-danthrusate are suitable)

Typical doses	Codanthramer forte	Codanthrusate caps
10 mg morphine 4-hourly	5 mls	2
30 mg morphine 4-hourly	10 mls	4
90 mg morphine 4-hourly	15 mls	6

   (Start low and titrate up)

4. **Have I prescribed a double dose at 10.00 pm to avoid waking this
   patient at 2.00 am?**
   Safe for morphine doses up to 40 mg four-hourly.

5. **Have I prescribed an anti-emetic prn?**
   Haloperidol 1.5–3 mg is suitable.

6. **Review this patient every twenty-four hours (at least) to adjust the dose.**

7. **Once this patient is stable, convert to MST twelve-hourly.**

8. **If oral medication is contraindicated for this patient, use subcutaneous
   diamorphine (one third oral morphine dose).**

Morphine information

1. What is morphine?

It is made from opium poppies. It works as a strong painkiller and when used correctly in the right sort of dose there is no evidence that it either shortens or prolongs life.

2. How is morpine taken?

These are two common ways of taking morphine:

i)   As slow-acting morphine
     This is usually as slow release tablets which last twelve hours. Examples of these are MST continuous and Oramorph SR. They come in a variety of strengths from 5mg through to 200mg. Because they last for twelve hours, they need to be taken at twelve-hourly intervals, eg. 9.00am and 9.00pm or 10.00am and 10.00pm. They are not suitable for a sudden sharp pain in between. Slow-release morphine is also available in liquid form.

ii) Fast-acting morphine
     This comes as a liquid (Oramorph®) or as tablets (Sevredol®). Again, a variety of strengths may be prescribed. It starts to work within half to one hour of being taken and lasts for four hours. Fast-acting morphine is suitable for sudden pain despite your regular painkillers (breakthrough pain).

> The name of my slow-release morphine is: ....
> My present dose is: ....
> If I have pain in between I can take: ....

3. Does taking morphine mean I am near the end of the road?

Morphine is a strong painkiller. Doctors and nurses use it when there is strong pain. It can be administered after a serious accident or after an operation as well as being useful for cancer pain that is not relieved by more simple painkillers. The time to start using morphine is when the pain is bad enough.

4. Does morphine work for all pain?

No. Some pains are not helped by morphine. Your doctor will discuss this with you and sometimes it is necessary to take other painkillers at the same time as morphine.

5. Will I need larger and larger doses to control the pain?

Sometimes it is necessary to increase steadily the dose of morphine, particularly when beginning treatment, in order to work out the right level of painkiller for you. This is done slowly and steadily over a few days or someti mes a week or two. Further dose adjustment may be necessary as your illness goes on, but this only happens when the pain itself is getting worse. It does not mean that the morphine is losing its effect.

6.   What side-effects will I get?

i)   Constipation — although morphine is a good painkiller almost everybody who takes it gets constipated. You should make sure that your doctor routinely prescribes a good laxative which you need to take on a regular basis. This side-effect can also be helped by eating more fruit, vegetables, brown bread, bran-based breakfast cereals and drinking plenty of liquids.

ii)   Vomiting — about a third of people starting morphine can feel sickly or even vomit in the first week to ten days of treatment. Fortunately, the sickly feelings then usually disappear. If you are troubled by this side-effect an anti-sickness tablet can be prescribed for you to help you through the first week or two of treatment.

iii) Drowsiness — sometimes when starting morphine or after increasing the dose, people feel more sleepy or drowsy than usual for a day or two. For most people this quickly wears off. If it affects you, you should be careful not to drive or operate dangerous machinery. Less common side-effects when taking morphine are: unsteadiness, confusion, sweating, blurring of vision and a dry mouth.

7.   Will I become addicted to morphine?

When morphine is used as a painkiller, we know of no evidence that it causes addiction. If another treatment is possible that takes pain away we often find that we can reduce or even stop morphine. If you need to reduce or stop your morphine, it is wise to do this in discussion with a doctor as we like to reduce the dose gradually.

8.   What about driving?

Taking morphine does not automatically mean you cannot drive. You need to discuss driving with your doctor and common sense is needed. If your general alertness or concentration are poorer or if you are physically quite weak or ill, it may not be wise to drive. If your doctor says driving is OK, follow these general guidelines:
- ❖ do not drive in the dark or in bad conditions
- ❖ do not drink any alcohol before driving
- ❖ do not exhaust yourself by driving long distances.

9. Can I drink alcohol?

Yes. It is quite safe to drink alcohol while you are taking morphine. You may find that the combination of morphine and alcohol make you feel sleepy or drunk much sooner than usual, so it is sensible to drink much less than you are used to until you know what sort of effect it has on you.

West Cumbria Palliative Care Service
January 1997

2.5 Difficult pain problems

If pain control is difficult it is worth asking:

- is it the prescriber?
- is it the pain?
- is it the patient? (*Figure 2.5*).

Difficult pain — is it the prescriber?

⌘   Am I following basic prescribing guidelines?

⌘   Am I using the WHO analgesic ladder?

⌘   Have I titrated the morphine dose up individually for this patient according to clinical response?

⌘   Have I used appropriate formulations of morphine at the correct dose and the correct dosing interval?

⌘   Have I used co-analgesics and other interventions appropriately?

Difficult pain — is it the patient?

⌘   Is my patient taking the medication?

⌘   Are there fears/concerns or differing perceptions/priorities we have not recognized and addressed?

⌘   Does this pain have a significant psychosocial or spiritual component?

⌘   Is it worse when certain family members are there?

⌘   Is there co-existing depression?

⌘   Is there a lot of fear?

Difficult pain — is it the pain?

⌘   Is this a genuinely difficult pain?

⌘   Common examples of difficult pain are pancreatic pain, nerve pain and incident pain.

⌘   If so, have I discussed my approach with the specialist palliative care service?

Figure 2.5: Checklist for pain that is difficult to manage

2.6 Pain occurring despite regular background analgesia: breakthrough, incident and end-of-dose pain

Pain occurring despite regular background analgesia is commonly referred to as 'breakthrough' pain. It helps to be clear what is happening for the patient.

Breakthrough pain

The patient is taking long-acting analgesia, but continues to experience pain, episodically or continuously with no obvious precipitant. This occurs for two reasons: the pain is only partially opioid-sensitive; or the dose of long-acting opioid is too small. First, reassess the pain. Is it likely to be an opioid-sensitive pain? (See *Table 2.1.2. Interventions for the five common pain patterns, p. 11*).

⌘ Is the patient getting additional relief with IR opioid doses? (This helps confirm opioid sensitivity.) If so, increase the MR opioid by 30–50%. Remember to increase the dose of IR opioid to one-sixth of the new twenty-four-hour MR opioid dose.

⌘ Is it likely to be only partially opioid sensitive? Add in an appropriate co-analgesic (see *Table 2.11.1. Guidance for using co-analgesics*). Consider other interventions, such as radiotherapy for bone pain.

Incident pain

The patient experiences pain in specific situations only. Common situations in clinical practice are:

• weight-bearing pain in the presence of skeletal metastases
• movement-induced pain, particularly during personal nursing care in the bed-bound patient
• pain during painful procedures, such as dressing changes.

Incident pain is characterized by its rapid onset within seconds of the pain-provoking stimulus and its short duration. It usually settles within an hour or less of cessation of the painful stimulus.

The ideal analgesic in this situation is of **rapid onset and short duration**. Treatment options for incident pain are:

⌘ To use the usual IR opioid an hour before the painful procedure or anticipated painful activity. If the pain is intense, the dose can be increased in 30–50% increments until pain is controlled or limited by side-effects. For painful procedures in a bed-bound patient, the addition of midazolam 5–10 mg subcutaneously as a single dose can provide useful short-acting sedation.

⌘ If the usual IR opioid is morphine, a concentrated liquid formulation (20 mg/ml) can be prescribed in a bottle with calibrated dropper ('Oramorph® concentrated solution'). This allows small volumes of liquid to be administered, which can be held in the mouth to allow buccal absorption and rapid onset of action.

⌘ A diamorphine tablet (10 mg strength) can be dissolved sublingually, works within minutes and lasts up to four hours.

⌘ Oral transmucosal fentanyl citrate. Buccal lozenges on plastic sticks come in 200, 400, 600, 800, 1200 and 1600 μg lozenge strengths, which can be used up to four times a day. The lozenge strength is **not** related to the regular opioid dose. Start with 200 μg, which can be repeated after fifteen minutes if necessary. Titrate up in 200 μg steps to optimum tolerated dose. Do not exceed four doses in twenty-four hours.

For both breakthrough pain and incident pain, patients can gain much better relief if they and their carers are educated in the proactive use of analgesia. For example, simple advice about using short-acting analgesia prophylactically: 'Try taking your fast-acting morphine half an hour before you need to get dressed/wash/go shopping; expect it to make a difference for about four hours so use that time to do what you need without wearing yourself out'. It often helps patients and families to keep simple diaries of doses, time and effectiveness of additional analgesic doses. It gives them a sense of involvement and control over their pain, and is helpful to the doctor or nurse who comes to evaluate pain control, add up the average daily dose needed and translate it into an appropriate increment in the long-acting analgesic regimen.

End-of-dose pain

End-of-dose pain is pain occurring before the next dose of long-acting analgesia is due. It almost always means the dose of long-acting analgesia needs increasing, and this is the recommended action. Rarely, genuine rapid metabolisers have been described who may need a more frequent dosing schedule, such as eight-hourly administration for the twelve-hourly MR opioids or forty-eight-hourly patch changes for transdermal fentanyl.

Key points

❖ Pain occurring despite regular long-acting analgesia may be breakthrough pain, incident pain or end-of-dose pain.

❖ Breakthrough pain and end-of-dose pain will usually respond to an increase in the regular modified-release (MR) opioid.

❖ Sometimes breakthrough pain may occur because the pain is only partially responsive to morphine. The pain should be reassessed, and the role of co-analgesics and other interventions such as radiotherapy considered.

❖ Incident pain requires short-acting strong opioids of rapid onset. Buccal administration should be considered, and several drugs and formulations are suitable.

2.7 When to use alternatives to morphine

Morphine remains the 'gold standard' strong opioid analgesic for most patients. It is available in more formulations and strengths than any of the more recently introduced alternatives, giving great flexibility, particularly where low or high doses are needed.

Alternatives to morphine are worth considering in the following situations:

- patients with severe and uncontrollable morphine side-effects, such as confusion, hallucinations, drowsiness even at small doses, constipation or itch
- patients with renal failure
- patients afraid of morphine who are not able to rationalize their fears
- patients who are unable to swallow
- rarely as an 'opioid rotation' to attempt to improve overall analgesia where opioid-sensitive pain appears to be not responding to incremental morphine doses.

What are the alternatives?

Alternatives to morphine are strong (step 3) opioids, which fall into two main groups: oral preparations and transdermal fentanyl (see *Figure 2.7.1*).

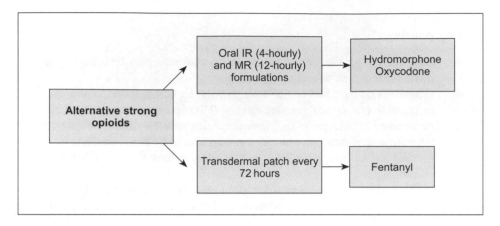

**Figure 2.7.1: Alternative strong opioids that can replace morphine.
IR=immediate release; MR=modified release**

Alternative strong opioids — oral preparations

There are two main alternative oral preparations — oxycodone and hydromorphone. Both come as IR formulations lasting four hours, which are suitable for dose titration or breakthrough pain, or as MR formulations lasting twelve hours, which are suitable for background pain relief.

The basic prescribing rules are similar to those for morphine:

- do not use two strong opioids if one will do (conversions get complicated)
- check doses carefully, referring to *Table 2.7.1* as a double check
- use the 30–50% rule for dose increments, rounding to the nearest tablet or capsule strength
- remember ABC (anti-emetic, breakthrough pain and constipation) and prescribe prophylactically
- prescribe breakthrough doses of one-sixth the total twenty-four-hour dose
- discuss or get advice from your local specialist palliative care team if you are unsure, or want to check anything
- plan proactively for how you will manage analgesia once the patient becomes unable to take oral medication
- not everyone is familiar with these drugs. Leave written information in the home for the patient, the rest of the practice team and the out-of-hours service (see *Figures 2.7.2* and *2.7.3* for examples of written information).

Once the patient becomes unable to take oral medication because death is near, the way forward will depend on why the alternative analgesic was chosen. Hydromorphone is available as a parenteral preparation suitable for subcutaneous administration, which currently needs pre-ordering on a named-patient basis from Martindales pharmaceuticals. A parenteral oxycodone preparation suitable for subcutaneous administration has recently been made available, but may not be routinely stocked by retail pharmacists. If the patient has a serious contraindication to morphine, this will need planning with your local pharmacy and possibly your local specialist team.

Many patients on alternative strong opioids for less serious indications will tolerate diamorphine through the last days of life. The conversion needs to be done with care, and *Table 2.7.1* will enable a rough check of its accuracy. Discuss with your local specialist team in advance if you are unsure.

Table 2.7.1: Approximate opioid equivalents

IR morphine (4-hourly)	MR morphine (12-hourly)	S/C diamorphine (24 hours)	IR hydro-morphone (4-hourly)	MR hydro-morphone (12-hourly)	IR oxycodone (4-hourly)	MR oxycodone (12-hourly)	Fentanyl μg/hourly patches
5	15	10	—	2	2.5	10	25
10	30	20	1.3	4	5	10	25
15	45	30	—	6	7.5	20	25
20	60	40	2.6	8	10	30	25
30	90	60	3.9	12	15	40	50
40	120	80	5.2	16	20	60	75
60	180	120	7.8	24	30	90	100
100	300	200	13	40	50	150	200
200	600	400	26	80	100	300	400
1	X 3	X 2	1/7.5	X 2/5	1/z	MST/2	Diamorphine mg/24 hours

IR = immediate relief (immediate or fast release); SC = subcutaneous; MR = modified relief (modified-release formulations)
All MR formulations on this chart are 12-hourly
Conversions are approximate; they are designed as a cross-check for safety, not as an accurate conversion tool
All patients on MR medication need IR medication for breakthrough pain and dose titration
Patients on fentanyl patches should be prescribed the appropriate dose of IR morphine, unless there are contraindications to morphine. In this situation, IR hydromorphone can be used instead
When patients on fentanyl need a syringe driver, the usual practice is to continue the fentanyl using an appropriate diamorphine increment (ie. equivalent to 30–50% fentanyl dose) in the syringe driver

Reproduced with kind permission from Eileen Palmer, West Cumbria Palliative Care Service, 2005

Dear...

Your patient .... has been discharged home on hydromorphone (Palladone).

Hydromorphone is a strong opioid that is occasionally used as an alternative to morphine. The range of side effects are similar, with constipation being the commonest. Like morphine, hydromorphone comes in slow-release (12-hourly) and immediate-release (4-hourly) formulations. The range of capsule strengths and morphine equivalents are tabulated below.

Your patient is currently on hydromorphone MR .... 12-hourly (Palladone).

If they have breakthrough pain they can take:

Hydromorphone IR ....

The dose of hydromorphone MR can be titrated up in 30–50% increments (as with MST).

The dose of hydromorphone IR is approximately 1/6 of the total daily dose (as with Oramorph).

If you have any queries please telephone:..

Hydromorphone capsule strengths and morphine equivalents			
Morphine		**Hydromorphone**	
MST 12-hourly (mg)	Oramorph for breakthrough (mg)	Hydromorphone SR 12-hourly (mg)	Hydromorphone IR for breakthrough (mg)
15	5	2	1.3
30	10	4	1.3
60	20	8	2.6
120	40	16	5.2
180	60	24	7.8

Figure 2.7.2: Example of a hydromorphone information leaflet issued by the Ennerdale Palliative Care Unit, West Cumberland Hospital, Whitehaven, Cumbria

Dear...

Your patient .... has been discharged home on oxycodone MR (Oxycontin®).

Oxycodone is a strong opioid that is occasionally used as an alternative to morphine. The range of side effects are similar, with constipation being the commonest. Like morphine, oxycodone comes in slow-release (12-hourly) and immediate-release (4-hourly) formulations. The range of tablet strengths and morphine equivalents are tabulated below.

Your patient is currently on Oxycodone MR .... 12-hourly (Oxycontin®).

If they have breakthrough pain they can take:

Oxycodone IR (Oxynorm®) ....

The dose of Oxycodone MR can be titrated up in 30–50% increments (as with MST).

The dose of Oxycodone IR is approximately one-sixth of the total daily dose (as with Oramorph®).

Oxycodone capsule strengths and morphine equivalents			
Morphine		**Oxycodone**	
MST 12-hourly (mg)	Oramorph for breakthrough (mg)	Oxycodone MR 12-hourly (mg)	Oxycodone IR for breakthrough (mg)
20	5	10	5
40	10	20	5
80	30	40	15
160	60	80	30
		MR capsules available as 10 mg, 20 mg, 40 mg, 80 mg strengths	IR capsules available as 5 mg, 10 mg, 20 mg strengths

Figure 2.7.3: Example of an oxycodone information leaflet issued by the Ennerdale Palliative Care Unit, West Cumberland Hospital, Whitehaven, Cumbria

Alternative strong opioids — transdermal fentanyl

Fentanyl is a strong (step 3) opioid, which is lipid soluble, making it suitable for transdermal administration. This follows a different pattern of absorption and takes skill to use well. *It is not suitable alone for the rapid control of severe pain.* It may take thirty-six to forty-eight hours to achieve steady-state plasma concentrations after the patch has been applied, and there is considerable inter-individual variability. If for any reason the patch needs to be removed, significant plasma levels may persist for twenty-four hours or more. Fentanyl is *slow* to build up and *slow* to clear.

The prescribing rules for fentanyl are consequently different to all the other strong opioids:

- reserve for situations where rapid dose adjustments are unlikely to be necessary
- patch strengths available are 25 μg/hour, 50 μg/hour, 75 μg/hour and 100 μg/hour
- to quickly convert to a fentanyl patch from oral morphine, calculate the twenty-four-hour morphine dose in mg and divide by three
- prescribe the nearest equivalent patch strength in μg/hour
- to transfer from a twelve-hourly MR opioid, apply the closest equivalent strength of fentanyl patch (see *Table 2.7.1*) at the same time the last twelve-hourly dose is given
- remember to instruct the patient to discontinue their MR opioid after this
- encourage the patient to use additional doses of IR opioid liberally during the first three days as the plasma fentanyl level builds up (see *Table 2.7.2*)
- if the patient still needs more than two additional doses of IR opioid twenty-four hours after the first three days, increase the patch strength by 25 μg/hour
- if the patient has been on prophylactic laxatives, halve the dose of laxative and monitor
- discuss or get advice from your local specialist palliative care team if you are unsure, or want to check anything
- plan proactively for how you will manage analgesia once the patient becomes unable to take oral medication (see below)
- not everyone is familiar with this drug. Leave written information in the home for the patient, the rest of the practice team and the out-of-hours service.

Table 2.7.2: IR opioid doses to use with transdermal fentanyl

IR opioid	IR dose
IR morphine	Half the fentanyl patch strength as IR morphine in mg (eg. for 25 µg/hour patch strength give IR morphine 10–15 mg as required)
IR hydromorphone	Approximately one-fifteenth of the fentanyl patch strength as IR hydromorphone in mg (eg. for 25 µg/hour patch strength give IR hydromorphone 1.3 mg)*
IR oxycodone	One-quarter the fentanyl patch strength as IR oxycodone in mg (eg. for 25 µg/hour patch strength give IR oxycodone 5 mg)*
Oral transmucosal fentanyl citrate (OTFC)	No relationship to fentanyl patch strength. Lozenge strength **not** related to regular opioid dose. Start with 200 µg; repeat after 15 minutes if necessary. Titrate up in 200 µg steps to optimum tolerated dose. Do not exceed four doses in 24 hours

*For all these conversions the practicality of the range of tablet strengths available may mean a slight adjustment to the closest reasonably administered dose. Double-check your conversion if necessary in *Table 2.7.1*

Using fentanyl in the dying patient

Sometimes there is confusion about how best to manage a patient who has been using fentanyl patches for pain control, but who is dying and can no longer take oral medication for breakthrough pain.

These guidelines are intended to clarify and simplify good practice:

- *Continue* to change the fentanyl patch every three days.
- If additional analgesia is necessary, subcutaneous diamorphine should be given. This can be administered in a syringe driver with additional four-hourly subcutaneous injections available for immediate relief of breakthrough pain. Appropriate doses are given in *Table 2.7.3*.

Table 2.7.3: Dosage guidelines for use of fentanyl patch with subcutaneous diamorphine*

Fentanyl patch strength (µg/hour)	Diamorphine (mg/24 hours subcutaneously)	Diamorphine (mg/4 hours subcutaneously for breakthrough pain)
25	15	5–10
50	30	5–10
75	40	10–20
100	60	20–30
200	100	25–50

*The diamorphine is given in addition to the fentanyl patch

- The fentanyl patch should only be discontinued in exceptional circumstances by practitioners with a good working knowledge of the pharmacodynamics of fentanyl. Many practitioners may prefer to seek expert advice first from a member of the palliative care team. (See *Table 2.7.4, opposite.*)

2.8 Which alternative strong opioid should I choose?

Most of us are familiar with the use of morphine, but few of us have experience of all the alternative strong opioids; use the one you have greatest familiarity and skill with. If you have a good working knowledge of the use of all of them, choices can also be guided by the reason for selecting an alternative to morphine (see *Table 2.8.1, p. 36*).

2.9 Pain that does not respond well to morphine

Not all pain responds well to morphine. If you are not seeing some sign of incremental pain relief after increasing the morphine dose to the limits of the patient's tolerance, consider the following:

- review the diagnosis of the cause of the pain
- should you be adding in co-analgesics? For example, a non-steroidal anti-inflammatory drug for bone pain, or an antidepressant and/or

anticonvulsant for nerve pain (see co-analgesics [*Section 2.11*] and interventions for different pain patterns [*Table 2.1.2, p. 11*])
- are there appropriate non-drug interventions you could try? (see below)
- occasionally, switching patients from one strong opioid to another can enhance pain relief. This is sometimes called opioid rotation. Unless you have good familiarity with the drugs concerned, you may wish to discuss this with a specialist palliative care team first
- is this 'total pain?'

Table 2.7.4: A brief guide to alternative strong opioids

Drug	Strength	Frequency	Comments
Buprenorphine	200 µg tablets 400 µg tablets 300 µg injection	8-hourly 8-hourly 8-hourly	Tablets can be given sublingually. Partial morphine antagonist — do not use with other opioids. Analgesic ceiling at 3–5 mg/day equivalent to 180–300 mg morphine
Hydromorphone	Fast-release (IR) - 1.3 mg capsules - 2.6 mg capsules Modified-release (MR) - 2 mg capsules - 4 mg capsules - 8 mg capsules - 16 mg capsules - 24 mg capsules	 4-hourly 4-hourly 12-hourly 12-hourly 12-hourly 12-hourly 12-hourly	Equivalent to: - 10 mg morphine - 20 mg morphine Equivalent to: - 15 mg morphine - 30 mg morphine - 60 mg morphine - 120 mg morphine - 180 mg morphine
Oxycodone	Fast-release (IR) - 5 mg capsules - 10 mg capsules - 20 mg capsules Slow-release (MR) - 10 mg capsules - 20 mg capsules - 40 mg capsules - 80 mg capsules	 4-hourly 4-hourly 4-hourly 12-hourly 12-hourly 12-hourly 12-hourly	Equivalent to: - 10 mg morphine - 20 mg morphine - 40 mg morphine Equivalent to: - 20 mg morphine - 40 mg morphine - 80 mg morphine - 160 mg morphine
Methadone	5 mg tablet Linctus 2 mg/5 ml Injection 10 mg/ml	8–12-hourly	Mixed mu/delta-agonist NMDA receptor antagonist. Occasionally good for morphine-resistant pain. Half-life 8–80 hours. Titrate 3-hourly as necessary for up to 6 days, then a twice-daily dose
Fentanyl	 25 µg/hour patch 50 µg/hour patch 75 µg/hour patch 100 µg/hour patch	 Every 3 days Every 3 days Every 3 days Every 3 days	Equivalent to: - approximately 15 mg morphine 4-hourly - 30 mg morphine 4-hourly - 40 mg morphine 4-hourly - 60 mg morphine 4-hourly Takes 3–23 hours to reach effective analgesic level, 36–48 hours to reach steady state. *Always prescribe a fast-acting opioid for breakthrough pain*

Table 2.8.1: Guidelines to prescribing a strong opioid other than morphine

Reason for selecting an alternative to morphine	Potential choices
Cognitive side effects; confusion/drowsiness even at small doses	Hydromorphone Oxycodone Fentanyl
Intractable constipation despite optimal laxatives	Fentanyl
Itch	Oxycodone
Difficulty swallowing	Hydromorphone* MST granules Fentanyl
Fear of morphine	Any
Renal failure	Hydromorphone Oxycodone Fentanyl

*Break capsules open and sprinkle onto/into soft food

2.10 Total pain

At some point, pain stops being pain, stops being identifiable; it becomes a state of being. I couldn't have said whether I was in pain or not. I certainly didn't have a vocabulary to describe it or even locate it. I just knew I was suffering in the most unusual, unreal manner. It just seemed that everything was pain.

Patient with cancer.

Total pain is physical pain, complicated and exacerbated by fear. It is a situation of great suffering and anguish for the patient and for everyone around the patient. It is a palliative care emergency. It is a crisis at every level:

⌘ **Physical** — uncontrolled pain.
⌘ **Emotional** — anxiety, sadness, anger, fear.
⌘ **Social** — severe carer strain, loss of confidence, fear, distress.
⌘ **Spiritual** — anguish, suffering, hopelessness, meaningless.

It requires intervention at every level and the skill and experience of a multiprofessional team. Unless the emotional and spiritual aspects are addressed, physical pain control can be impossible.

2.11 Co-analgesics

Cancer pain can be:

- morphine-responsive
- partly morphine-responsive
- morphine-resistant.

Co-analgesics may either complement or replace conventional analgesics where pain is not completely responsive to morphine (see *Table 2.11.1*).

Table 2.11.1: Guidance for using co-analgesics

Drug	Some uses	Some problems
Non-steroidal anti-inflammatory drugs (eg. naproxen 500 mg twice-daily, diclofenac 50 mg three times a day)	Bone pain Soft-tissue pain	Dyspepsia Fluid retention and oedema Gastrointestinal bleeding, peptic ulcers, wheezing and rashes
Steroids (eg. prednisolone, dexamethasone 4–16 mg daily)	Nerve compression pain Headache of raised intracranial pressure Spinal cord compression Metastatic arthralgia Hepatomegaly	Oral thrush Ankle oedema Moon face Agitation Psychosis Proximal myopathy Gastritis/peptic ulcer Diabetes
Tricyclic antidepressants, eg. amitryptiline 25 mg once daily, dothiepin 25 mg once daily, venlafaxine	Nerve destruction pain (burning, parasthesiae)	Sedation Dry mouth Constipation Retention of urine Dizziness/confusion
Anticonvulsants, eg. carbamazepine, sodium valproate 400 mg–1 g daily, gabapentin 100–300 mg three times a day	Nerve compression and destruction pain (jabbing, stabbing)	Drowsiness/ataxia Nausea Rashes Hepatitis
Muscle relaxants, eg. diazepam, baclofen	Muscle spasm	Drowsiness
Antibiotics	Infection	

2.12. Diamorphine prescribing at the end of life

Diamorphine is frequently prescribed in the last few days of life. In the wake of the Shipman trial, it is even more important for patients, families and the GP and primary healthcare team to be confident that diamorphine is being prescribed correctly. This means prescribing appropriate and defensible doses for appropriate and documented indications. Clear discussion with the patient and the family about the indication and dosage is vital.

Diamorphine is primarily a strong analgesic. It is a cough suppressant and, in the absence of pain, a respiratory sedative. This side effect can be used to relieve distressing breathlessness at the end of life.

Diamorphine is *not* a strong sedative. It is generally unsuitable for terminal agitation, anguish or distress, and if used inappropriately it may cause or exacerbate these problems. In the absence of pain or in excessive doses, diamorphine can cause nightmares, hallucinations, sweating, confusion and myoclonic jerks. If a patient needs sedation, benzodiazepines are a better choice. *Table 2.12.1* outlines diamorphine prescribing at the end of life.

Sometimes if a patient is in severe pain and near death, it can be tempting to put a much larger dose of diamorphine in the syringe driver. This is unsatisfactory for two reasons:

- diamorphine from a syringe driver takes about four hours to build up to a steady plasma level, so is not quick enough
- it is difficult to guess the correct dose, particularly in a patient who has not had opioids before. Too little and the patient is still in pain; too much and the patient may die from an opioid overdose. With severe pain, it is better to prescribe a safe and defensible dose of diamorphine in the syringe driver, following the guidance above, and to give 'as required' doses every hour or so to quickly gain both pain control and a sense of correct twenty-four-hour requirement.

Table 2.12.1: Diamorphine regimen at the end of a patient's life

Clinical situation at the end of life	Subcutaneous diamorphine dose over 24 hours	'As required' subcutaneous diamorphine dose
No previous opioid No pain	Not indicated	2.5–5 mg s/c as required
No previous opioid In pain	20 mg/24 hours (halve dose if >70 years old or frail)	2.5–5 mg s/c as required
On oral morphine No pain	Oral morphine dose in mg/24 hours divided by three	One-sixth of 24-hour dose of diamorphine in mg s/c as required
On oral morphine In pain	Oral morphine dose in mg/24 hours divided by two	One-sixth of 24-hour dose of diamorphine in mg s/c as required

2.13 Non-drug treatments of pain

Explanation

A vital part of all pain management is explanation of the reason for the pain and the rationale for the management plan. This will reduce fear and anxiety and increase trust and partnership (which will also improve compliance).

Radiotherapy

⌘ Always consider radiotherapy for painful bone metastases provided the patient has a prognosis of at least six weeks.
⌘ Consider for painful skin metastases, fungating tumours, painful mass lesions, chest wall pain from carcinoma of the bronchus and nerve pain from spinal metastases.
⌘ If in doubt discuss with an oncologist.

Surgical stabilization of bones

⌘ An unstable spine or lytic lesions in long bones can give severe pain control problems.
⌘ If >50% bone loss, the patient is also at risk of pathological fracture.
⌘ Minimize weight bearing and discuss with an orthopaedic surgeon.

Acupuncture

⌘ This may help a significant number of cancer pain syndromes to some degree.
⌘ Needs availability of a local skilled practitioner.
⌘ Some physiotherapists and a number of doctors have acupuncture training.
⌘ Duration of pain relief short, necessitating multiple treatments.
⌘ Invasive, but simple and safe.

Transcutaneous electrical nerve stimulation

⌘ Benefit in a wide variety of painful conditions, but unpredictable who will respond.
⌘ Needs availability of local skilled practitioner (and loan system for machines).
⌘ Often available through pain clinics or physiotherapy departments.
⌘ Efficacy diminishes with time.
⌘ Patients need instruction and support in use.
⌘ Needs to be used up to three times a day; compliance may be poor.
⌘ Simple and safe.
⌘ May be better for limb pain than trunk pain.

Heat/cold

⌘ Icepacks and hot water bottles are widely used to ease aches and pains.
⌘ Hot packs and cold packs (reusable gel packs) provide another alternative.
⌘ May relieve muscle spasm, back pain, joint pains secondary to immobility.
⌘ A cold pack can relieve non-specific headache.
⌘ Heat may help abdominal colic.

Modification of behaviour

⌘ Distraction, either by absorption in activities of interest or through specific interventions such as listening to music or relaxation tapes through earphones, may reduce pain perception. Attendance at a day hospice may provide this.
⌘ Hypnotherapy or taught self-hypnosis can sometimes help modify the pain experience. It can also reduce associated anxiety.
⌘ Avoiding painful activity. For skeletal metastases in weight-bearing areas this may mean a walking aid, a wheelchair or occasionally even bedrest and catheterization, depending on the success of other interventions.

Positioning

⌘ Support or protect painful areas with pillows/cushions/cradles.

⌘ District nurses may wish to involve the physiotherapist or occupational therapist for advice and support if moving and handling is painful.

Anaesthetic interventions

⌘ These may help about 8% of cancer patients with pain.
⌘ Coeliac or splanchnic nerve blocks are useful for pancreatic pain or severe upper gastrointestinal pain.
⌘ Lumbar sympathetic blocks may relieve intractable tenesmus or rectal pain.
⌘ Intercostal nerve blocks can sometimes help unilateral chest wall pain.
⌘ Trigger point injections of local anaesthetic may relieve myofascial pain.
⌘ A skilled anaesthetist may be able to place a cannula over the brachial plexus or femoral nerve, relieving intractable limb pain.
⌘ Spinal opioids help with some intractable pain syndromes.
⌘ Discuss with a pain anaesthetist.

Key points

❖ Morphine is the gold standard for most patients.
❖ Oral alternatives to morphine follow broadly similar prescribing rules to morphine.
❖ Fentanyl patches are used and prescribed differently.
❖ If prescribing an alternative to morphine, the prescriber needs a good working knowledge of safe prescribing practice for the drug and its approximate morphine equivalence.
❖ Not everyone is familiar with these drugs. Leave written information in the home for the patient, the rest of the practice team and the out-of-hours service.
❖ Discuss or get advice from your local specialist palliative care team if you are unsure or want to check anything.
❖ Plan proactively for how you will manage analgesia once the patient becomes unable to take oral medication.
❖ Consider the use of co-analgesics for pain that is not responding to morphine.
❖ Remember to look at non-drug interventions.

2.14: A brief guide to alternative methods of drug administration

Patients are not always able to take oral medication. The syringe driver has been such an important advance as a drug delivery system for those patients that alternatives do not always spring readily to mind. Syringe drivers are not always appropriate. A crisis may arise when one is not readily available. The patient may not wish to carry the apparatus around, or may dislike the constant reminder of illness. The patient may wish to travel and be independent of the need for daily nursing checks for a few days. Injections may be contraindicated because of coagulation defects or severe immunosuppresion. What alternatives are there?

⌘ Rectal administration. A good range of analgesics, anti-emetics and sedatives can be administered rectally.
⌘ Sublingual administration (also buccal preparations) (*Table 2.14.1*).
⌘ Transdermal administration. Transdermal fentanyl is an alternative strong opioid to morphine. It is suitable for patients with stable pain relief requirements. Transdermal hyoscine is well established. (*Table 2.14.2*).

Table 2.14.1: Sublingual and buccal preparations*

Drug	Route	Comments
Analgesics		
Aspirin 500 mg (Palaprim forte)	2 tablets, four times a day, chewed or sucked	Care with gastrointestinal side-effects
Buprenorphine 200 µg, 400 µg (Temgesic)	Sublingual, 8-hourly	Useful for opiate-sensitive pain. Possible dose 'ceiling' at about 3 mg per day. *Do not use at the same time as morphine* (antagonism)
Sevredol® 10 mg, 20 mg (morphine)	Buccal 4-hourly	Rapid onset within 5–15 minutes. Unpleasant taste
Oramorph® concentrated solution 100 mg/5 ml (morphine)	Buccal 4-hourly	Volume of administration *usually* sufficiently small to enable patient to hold solution in the mouth allowing buccal absorption. Comes with dropper
Fentanyl lozenges (oral transmucosal fentanyl citrate or OTFC)	Buccal up to four times a day 200, 400, 600, 800, 1200, 1600 µg lozenge strengths	Lozenge strength *not* related to regular opioid dose. Start with 200 µg, repeat after 15 minutes if necessary. Titrate up in 200 µg steps to optimum tolerated dose. Do not exceed 4 doses in 24 hours

Table 2.14.1 cont: Sublingual and buccal preparations*

Anti-emetics

Buccastem® (prochlorperazine)	Buccal 1–2 twice-daily	Acts on CTZ. More sedating and probably less effective than haloperidol but useful in this formulation
Hyoscine — oral 0.3 mg (Kwells)	Suck in mouth	Can also use injectable hyoscine sublingually. Useful for vomiting from intestinal obstruction

Anxiolytics

Lorazepam	Buccal or sublingual 0.5–2 mg	Rapid onset. Useful for panic, especially respiratory panic

*Rapid onset of action (within 5–15 minutes). Patients need careful explanation of use. If the mouth is dry, advise the patient to moisten it with a sip of water before use. CTZ=chemoreceptor trigger zone in the floor of the fourth ventricle of the brain

Table 2.14.2: Transdermal preparation

Drug	Route	Comments
Fentanyl	Apply to flat, dry, hairless skin on the upper body every 72 hours; 25 µg/h, 50 µg/h, 75 µg/h, 100 µg/h patch strengths available	• Suitable for stable pain • Ensure patient has short-acting strong opioid for breakthrough pain • Slow onset (36–48 hours) and long elimination half-life (24 hours)
ScopadermTTS Hyoscine 1 mg	Transdermal patch 1mg/72h	• Dries secretions, eg. sialorrhoea, dysphagia, 'death rattle' • Antiemetic, particularly with intestinal obstruction. Sedating. Paradoxical confusion/agitation in about 10%

2.15: A brief guide to emergency drugs in palliative care

Anticipation of problems is an important part of good palliative care. Most emergencies that arise can be dealt with by a relatively small core of drugs (*Table 2.15.1*). Experience dictates that many emergencies arise at night or at weekends, when it may be difficult to get hold of medications quickly. It is well worth considering keeping these drugs in readily available places, such as the patient's house or the doctor's bag.

Table 2.15.1: Drugs used for emergency palliative care

Drug	Strength	Indications
Diamorphine injection	Proportional to patient's regular analgesia. A dose for breakthrough pain should be 50–100% of the patient's usual 4-hourly diamorphine dose (for a syringe driver running over 24 hours, divide by 6). To convert from oral morphine (mg) to parenteral diamorphine (mg) divide by 3	Breakthrough pain Breathlessness
Dexamethasone injection	12–24 mg intravenously	Suspected: – spinal cord compression (vertebral pain, radicular pain, later sensory changes, motor weakness progressing to sphincter disturbance) – laryngeal or tracheal obstruction (stridor) – SVC obstruction (oedema, prominent veins, dusky colour to face and arms, headache) All need to be followed by urgent radiotherapy referral
Hyoscine hydrobromide 0.4 mg as required (0.4 mg injection)	Maximum 2.4 mg/24 hours	Dries up secretions Antiemetic Sedating
Haloperidol 5 mg injection	3 mg subcutaneously for vomiting 10 mg subcutaneously as an antipsychotic, repeated hourly if necessary up to 30 mg/24 hours	Antiemetic Agitation/restlessness (with evidence of hallucinations or paranoia)
Midazolam 10 mg injection	5–10 mg as a single dose 20–30 mg subcutaneously over 24 hours (can be titrated up to 40–60 mg if necessary)	Anxiety Agitation/restlessness without evidence of hallucinations) Anticonvulsant Sedation for catastrophic emergency, eg. major haemorrhage
or		
Diazepam injection (emulsion) 5 mg or rectal solution or suppositories	5–10 mg intravenously at a rate of <5 mg/minute 5–10 mg as a single dose rectally Repeat after 5 minutes if necessary	As above As above

References

American Pain Society (1992) *Principles of Analgesic Use in the Treatment of Cancer Pain*. 3rd edn. American Pain Society, Glenview, Illinois

Friedman DP (1990) Perspectives on the medical use of drugs of abuse. *J Pain Symptom Manage* **5**: S2–5

Portenoy RK (1995) Pharmacological management of cancer pain. *Sem Oncol* **22**: 112–120

World Health Organization (1990) *Cancer Pain Relief and Palliative Care*. Technical Report Series 804. WHO, Geneva

Bibliography

Clinical Guidelines Working Party (2003) *Guidance for Managing Cancer Pain in Adults*. 3rd edn. National Hospice for Hospice and Palliative Care: June

Morphine and alternative strong opioids in cancer pain: the EAPC recommendations. Expert Working Group of the Research Network of the European Association for Palliative Care (2001) Hanks *et al Br J Cancer* **84**(5): 587–93

Regnard C, Hockley J (2004) *A Guide to Symptom Relief in Palliative Care*. 5th edn. Radcliffe Medical Press, Oxford

Scottish Intercollegiate Guidelines Network (2000) *Control of Pain in Patients with Cancer*. SIGN, Royal College of Physicians of Edinburgh

Twycross R (1994) *Pain Relief in Advanced Cancer*. Churchill Livingstone, London

Twycross R, Wilcock A, Thorp S (2002) *Palliative Care Formulary*. 2nd edn. Radcliffe Medical Press, Oxford

Twycross R Wilcock A (2001) *Symptom Management in Advanced Cancer*. Radcliffe Medical Press, Oxford

3

Physical problems in palliative care A–Z

3.1 Anorexia (see also nutrition, *Chapter 4*)

Anorexia is an extremely common problem that is often overlooked. This problem can cause great distress to patients and their families. Calorie intake can be increased by the following (see also *Figure 3.1.1*):

⌘ Make a range of liquid food supplements available. These vary widely in taste, texture and palatability. Different ones suit different patients.

⌘ It can be helpful to persuade local pharmacists to stock 'taster packs' with different makes and flavours. Recipe books and leaflets are available from manufacturers, or practices can devise their own.

⌘ Menus can be simply enriched in protein and calories by using full-cream milk products, dried milk powder, cream and butter to enrich familiar and favourite recipes.

⌘ Alcohol in small amounts before a main meal is a traditional appetite stimulant, provided this is acceptable to the patient.

⌘ Dexamethasone 4 mg daily will stimulate appetite and wellbeing in a proportion of patients. It usually works within a week; if it does not make a difference after a week it should be stopped as it carries a significant burden of side-effects. Where it does work, benefit can be sustained for a number of weeks

⌘ Megestrol acetate 80–160 mg daily, increased to twice or three times a day, may have a longer acting effect on appetite and weight gain. It is more expensive.

Easy ways to boost your calorie intake

Fortified or double strength milk

This is very easy to make and can be used in many different foods.

To 1 pint of full cream milk add 2oz dried milk, eg. Marvel, mix well with a whisk or in a liquidiser/food processor.

This can be used to replace ordinary milk in drinks (tea, coffee, milk shakes), dried or condensed soups, sauces, instant mash potato, on cereal or to make up puddings, such as Angel Delight, custard, etc.

If you are concerned about your fat intake, you could use 1 pint of skimmed milk with 3oz of skimmed milk powder. This version is a little lower in calories but still much better than unfortified milk.

> Dietitian.......................
> Date.............................
> Dietetic Department
> West Cumberland Hospital
> Whitehaven CA28 8JG

Grated cheese

This is always useful and can be added to a large variety of foods, including soup, mashed potato, baked potato, scrambled egg, omelette, savoury egg custard and any savoury sauces used with pasta, fish, etc.

Note: it is probably wiser to use a crumbly cheese (eg. Cheshire type) to top shepherd's pie/lasagne etc, as some cheeses may become stringy and difficult to swallow when melted.

Evaporated milk/double cream

Mix dried soups, sauces, instant mashed potato, scrambled egg, savoury egg custard and any savoury sauces used for pasta, fish, etc. with evaporated milk or cream, or a mixture of the two. They can also be used very well with sweet foods, eg. custard, added to yoghurt, used with sponge cake and added to breakfast cereals.

Butter/margarine/mayonnaise/salad cream
Another good source of calories, they can be added to potatoes, mashed boiled or baked. Also, butter or margarine add calories to hot vegetables, eg. buttered carrots or corn on the cob. Spread butter or margarine generously on bread or toast. Mix fish (eg. tuna) or grated cheese with mayonnaise or salad cream to boost the calorie content.

Honey/jams/marmalade/sugars/syrup
Any of these can be added to foods to boost your calorie intake. Put a thick layer of marmalade on toast for your breakfast. Add a couple of teaspoons of jam to milk puddings. Honey can be added to hot drinks, eg. honey and lemon or mixed with a little hot whisky as a nightcap (check with your doctor in case you are not allowed alcohol). Extra syrup can be added into cooking, try using 1½ times the quantity stated in the recipe for things such as flapjacks or add an extra spoonful of syrup to tinned syrup sponge. Sugar itself is easily included into many foods, eg. breakfast cereals, hot drinks such as tea and coffee. If you have a sweet tooth you could slice fresh fruit, eg. banana or strawberries and add a couple of teaspoons of sugar or drizzle with honey and add cream or Greek yoghurt. Drizzle honey or syrup over cereal or porridge.

Figure 3.1.1: Easy ways to boost your calorie intake. Reproduced by kind permission of the Dietetic Department, West Cumberland Hospital, West Cumbria Health Care NHS Trust

3.2 Ascites

Between 15–50% of patients with malignancy may develop ascites. It is classically associated with ovarian cancer, where it is said to occur in 30% of patients at presentation and over 60% by death.

Ascites presents as bloating and abdominal distension. It is detected clinically by the finding of flank dullness, shifting dullness and possibly a fluid thrill. It can be confirmed by ultrasound scan, which can also help localize the best site for drainage of a loculated collection.

Symptoms

- ✻ Relate to the pressure effect of the fluid.
- ✻ Abdominal distension, tightness, pain, restricted mobility.

⌘ Pressure on the stomach causing nausea, vomiting, reflux symptoms, early satiation, hiccoughs.

⌘ Pressure on the diaphragm causing dyspnoea.

Management

⌘ **Diuretics**. Provided these can be tolerated and renal function is adequate, prescribe spironolactone 100 mg/day. Increase by 100 mg every three days to obtain a response (weight loss 0.5–1 kg/day). Two-thirds of patients respond to 300 mg/day; maximum dose is 400 mg/day. If not responding, add in frusemide 40 mg/day. Monitor urea and electrolytes weekly; watch for dehydration at higher doses.

⌘ **Paracentesis**. Can give quick relief for the patient who is symptomatic. It rarely gives sustained benefit, and repeated paracenteses can lead to protein depletion.

3.3 Bowel obstruction

Typical symptoms of acute bowel obstruction taught in medical schools include gaseous distension, high-pitched bowel sounds, constipation and colic. Abdominal X-ray generally confirms the diagnosis, with distended loops of bowel and fluid levels on erect films. However, **in palliative care many bowel obstructions present subacutely, often just with vomiting**.

Step 1. Suspect

Have a high index of suspicion, especially with a history of:

• pelvic malignancy
• primary bowel cancer
• known peritoneal involvement, when combined with **a history of episodic vomiting over weeks or months**.

The underlying pathology is often multiple-site, small-bowel obstruction. Unlike acute obstruction, abdominal distension, colic and constipation do not invariably feature until a late stage, and plain abdominal X-rays may be normal. Diagnosis is then clinical.

Most bowel obstruction in palliative care can be managed medically with good symptom control. Traditional surgical interventions, such as nasogastric tubes and intravenous infusions, are avoided where possible. It is, however, important to screen out those patients who have single-site obstruction, which would respond well to surgery.

Step 2. Is it operable?

⌘ Is there evidence of a single-site block (colic, distension)?
⌘ Is there marked abdominal distension?
⌘ Are there two or more loops of bowel on erect X-ray (as opposed to multiple, small fluid levels)
⌘ Is there no evidence of a large abdominal tumour mass or massive ascites?
⌘ Is the patient's general condition good?
⌘ Does the patient wish surgery?

Discuss the situation with the surgeon or specialist palliative care colleagues if there is doubt.

Step 3. Medical management (see Table 3.2.1)

Table 3.2.1: Medical management for bowel obstruction[*]

Colic	Discontinue stimulant laxatives, eg. senna, co-danthramer Discontinue prokinetic drugs, eg. metoclopramide Start hyoscine butylbromide 60 mg/24 hours subcutaneously (Coeliac plexus block)
Abdominal pain	Diamorphine subcutaneously in a dose proportional to previous opiate requirement and pain level (Coeliac plexus block)
Vomiting	Haloperidol 5 mg/24 hours Cyclizine 100–150 mg/24 hours (in combination with haloperidol) If still nauseated/vomiting, seek advice from a specialist palliative care resource. Sometimes, low-dose levomepromazine (6.25–12.5 mg/24 hours) or a trial of an antisecretory such as hyoscine butylbromide 60 mg/24 hours or even octreotide 3–600 µg/24 hours may be suggested For high obstruction (above mid-jejunum), consider nasogastric tube Consider venting gastrostomy

*If symptoms are not resolving quickly with anti-emetics, anti-spasmodics and analgesics, many specialist palliative care services recommend a trial of dexamethasone 8 mg a day for a week, which for some patients can bring rapid relief

3.4 Breathlessness

Exclude treatable causes clinically

Common, potentially correctable causes of breathlessness are anaemia, bronchospasm, cardiac failure and pleural effusion. A basic assessment will include screening for anaemia clinically, checking the haemoglobin level and listening to the chest for clinical signs of bronchospasm, left ventricular failure or pleural effusion.

Provided the patient has a life expectancy of at least two weeks and symptoms are sufficient to warrant intervention, a short admission to drain a pleural effusion or transfuse can give useful palliation.

Bronchodilators (preferably nebulized) or diuretics can be tried if clinically indicated, even in the last few days of life.

• Hyoscine hydrobromide or glycopyrollate can be used if the main symptom is excessive respiratory secretions at the end of life (see *Table 6.6.2*).

Consider a chest X-ray

Even in the absence of clinical signs, a chest X-ray may indicate lung metastases, a small effusion, segmental or lobar collapse or lymphangitis carcinomatosis.

Segmental or lobar collapse secondary to occlusion of an airway can sometimes be reversed by intraluminal radiotherapy, laser treatment or stenting, and provided the patient is committed to further intervention is worth discussing with your local chest physician.

Breathlessness from primary or secondary lung cancer can sometimes be palliated with radiotherapy; discuss with your local clinical oncologist.

Breathlessness secondary to lymphangitis carcinomatosis can sometimes be relieved with steroids, for example dexamethasone 4 mg daily.

Reduce the sensation of breathlessness

Respiratory sedatives reduce the sensation of breathlessness, whatever the cause. The commonest and most useful group is the strong opioids. Immediate-release (IR) morphine 5–10 mg will give helpful palliation for several hours. Patients can be advised to use it before activity to improve exercise tolerance.

Real life example

Gill was forty-six years old and had metastatic breast cancer, which had invaded her lungs and pleura, producing increasing and incapacitating breathlessness. Initially she got good relief from intermittent drainage of her pleural effusions. As her pulmonary disease progressed, she found she was breathless on minimal exertion, even after her effusion had been drained. This made it almost impossible to shop, and she hated relinquishing this role. She tried IR morphine 10 mg as required. She found if she took 10 mg before getting in her husband's car, by the time she got to the local supermarket she had enough relief to push the trolley around.

As the breathlessness deteriorates, modified-release (MR) preparations of morphine can be used to give more continuous relief, and the dose can be titrated up in 30–50% steps as long as it is tolerated in a similar way to its use for pain.

When the patient becomes unable to take oral morphine, a subcutaneous infusion of an equivalent dose of diamorphine will continue to provide ease, particularly if the breathing becomes very laboured and distressing.

Reduce the fear of breathlessness

Breathlessness is almost always frightening. Common fears are of choking or of suffocation. When patients are asked, many will describe respiratory panic attacks, where fear and breathlessness sustain each other in an escalating and terrifying cycle in which the patient believes he or she will almost certainly die (*Figure 3.4.1*).

Information about the conscious control of breathlessness, relaxation exercises, breathing exercises and individual or group support programmes can be of immense value in giving patients back a sense of control.

Benzodiazepines are a second group of respiratory sedatives that come into their own in this situation. As well as

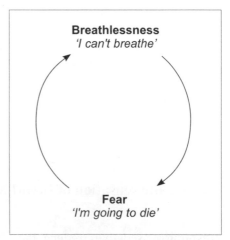

Figure 3.4.1: Terrifying circle of fear and breathlessness causes respiratory panic attacks

slowing and steadying the rate of breathing (by a central depressant action), they reduce fear and panic. Lorazepam 0.5 mg may be enough as a starting dose; for rapid relief it can be given sublingually. Always remember to ask the patient to moisten his or her mouth before sublingual administration. This is particularly important in this situation, as fear will make the mouth too dry for effective drug absorption otherwise. IR morphine liquid will suffice if administered just before the lorazepam. The lorazepam dose can be titrated up according to response. Most patients will respond to 0.5–2 mg twice or three times a day, as necessary.

As the patient deteriorates, subcutaneous midazolam can be used as an alternative, in a single dose of 5–10 mg or 10–30 mg over twenty-four hours via a syringe driver.

3.5 Constipation

There is no loneliness, shame and nightmare quite equal to constipation. For days on end all I would manage was blood and dribbles. I was scared to get off the toilet; scared I would have my own waste trickling down my legs. How many times did my children have to bang on the door in desperation to get me out of there? And then on the sixth day the sphincter would expand beyond the realms of known pain and there would be some result. No other experience has left me feeling so shamed, soiled, heartbroken, ineffectual, disappointed and dependant.

Cancer patient

Constipation is both preventable and treatable. It can be a miserable and undignified symptom. It warrants aggressive management. In one study of hospice inpatients, laxatives were needed by almost 90% of patients on opioids, and **also by two-thirds of patients on no opioids**.

Reduced food intake, weakness, debility and other constipating medications make constipation a common experience. It should be asked about as routinely as we would enquire about pain.

Self-help with breathlessness

Helping yourself with shortage of breath

For most people, feeling short of breath produces some natural responses that can make the problem even worse:

> Breathing with the shoulder and upper chest muscles. This is tiring and inefficient
> Breathing too quickly. This uses more energy and it causes shallow breathing, which is not so effective
> Fear, worry and panic. This causes muscles to tense and breathing to become even faster and shallower.

How to help yourself

> Find a comfortable position
> Practice gentle breathing:
> - try to pay attention to the feel of the breath as it enters the nose
> - breath gently in through the nose, then blow the breath out through the mouth
> - count to three as you breathe in, then count to six as you breathe out
>
> Relax the shoulders/upper chest. Allow these muscles to relax each time you breathe out. If this feels difficult, shrug your shoulders two or three times, then let your arms hang loosely and heavily at your sides. See if you can keep your shoulders relaxed as you breathe in, then out
> Breathe from your stomach. Place your hands on your stomach with the fingers just touching. As you breathe in, allow your stomach to expand, pushing your fingers apart a little. As you breathe out, allow it to relax and your fingers to touch again. Practice doing this slowly and deeply
> Calming the mind. Many people find this helps them feel more in control.

Practice the gentle breathing and try some of these calming techniques:

> - close your eyes and continue to count your breathing
> - say a calming phrase in your mind, eg. 'peace, calm, relax' or 'slow and deep, deep and slow'
> - imagine yourself in a beautiful and restful place. Try to imagine the scene in as much detail as you can
> - listen to music. Tape some of your favourite, most relaxing music
> - try a relaxation tape.

Modified from lecture notes and information leaflet from West Cumberland Hospital Breathlessness Clinic, West Cumbria Health Care NHS Trust

Prevention of constipation

⌘ Anticipate and ask all palliative care patients (not just those on opioids).
⌘ Laxatives should routinely be prescribed for patients starting strong opioids, and their effectiveness reviewed within three to five days (40% of patients will also require rectal measures).
⌘ Suitable laxatives include:
  • senna and docusate
  • senna and lactulose
  • co-danthramer or co-danthrusate
  • polyethylene glycol (one to three sachets daily).
⌘ The laxative dose should be titrated according to the response, both in regularity of bowel movement and in ease of defaecation.

Treatment of constipation

⌘ Exclude intestinal obstruction (see bowel obstruction, *Section 3.3*).
⌘ Either initiate or optimize a suitable oral laxative regimen (as above).
⌘ The laxative dose should be titrated according to the response, both in regularity of bowel movement and in ease of defaecation.
⌘ If there is no bowel motion after three days, proceed to rectal examination.
⌘ If the rectum is full, administer either a glycerin suppository and a bisacodyl suppository or a micro-enema.

Treatment of faecal impaction

For faecal impaction consider manual evacuation under sedation (diamorphine 5–10 mg; midazolam 5–10 mg subcutaneously half an hour before procedure) or polyethylene glycol (eight sachets daily for a maximum of three days). If using the latter, warn the patient to drink plenty, and have ready access to toilet facilities.

Constipation requires good teamwork between nurses, and between doctors and nurses. It is a symptom that can be managed more systematically with a protocol. An example of a bowel care protocol is given in *Figure 3.5.1*.

Bowel care protocol

On first assessment:

1. Record usual bowel habit and laxative use
2. Encourage fluids, fruit juices, fruit (including dried fruits), high-fibre cereals
3. Record bowel motions each day in bowel book/nursing care plan/ separate chart

If bowel habit normal: ensure all patients on regular opiates are prescribed a regular laxative, as below

If constipated: perform a rectal examination.

Is the rectum empty?

1. Exclude obstruction
2. Start laxative regimen

Is the rectum full?

1. Hard faeces
   – arachis oil enema at night
   – glycerin suppository and bisacodyl suppository
   – manual evacuation with sedation (gas/air or midazolam)
   – start or optimize laxative regimen
2. Soft faeces
   – micro-enema
   – start or optimize laxative regimen

Laxative regimen

Titrate up according to response.

Starting dose

● Co-danthramer 5–15 ml at night
● Co-danthrusate capsules 1–3 at night

Maximum dose

● Co-danthramer forte 15 ml twice a day
● Co-danthrusate capsules 3 capsules, three times a day

If ineffective at maximum dose, halve and add in a small bowel flusher, eg. lactulose 15–30 ml twice a day. Between 30–40% of patients will need regular rectal measures, despite regular laxatives by mouth. This is worth recognizing *early*, and a regimen of alternate-day suppositories or micro-enemas established.

Figure 3.5.1: An example of a bowel care protocol with a laxative regimen

Bibliography

Sykes NP (1994) Current approaches to the management of constipation. *Cancer Surv* **21**: 137–46

Sykes NP (1998) The relationship between opioid use and laxative use in terminally ill cancer patients. *Palliat Med* **12**(5): 375–82

Thorpe DM (2001) Management of opioid-induced constipation. *Curr Pain Headache Rep* **5**(3):237–40

3.6 Cough

Is this a dry cough?

⌘ Humidify the airway. Steam or nebulized saline can be used as necessary.
⌘ Simple linctus.
⌘ Codeine or pholcodine linctus.
⌘ Morphine 5–10 mg as required, which can be titrated up according to response in 30–50% increments (see morphine prescribing guidelines).

Methadone has been widely used as a cough suppressant in the past. It offers no advantages over morphine and is more likely to accumulate, particularly in the elderly, causing unacceptable toxicity.

Is this a moist cough?

⌘ Consider antibiotics if you suspect infection.
⌘ Liquefy secretions to improve expectoration. Steam inhalation or nebulized saline as necessary.
⌘ The physiotherapist may be able to advise patient and family on positioning.
⌘ Mucolytics, eg. carbocisteine.
⌘ Consider hyoscine transdermal patch or 0.3 mg sublingual if copious watery sputum.

3.7 Diarrhoea

Step 1. Differentiate

⌘ Diarrhoea.
⌘ Steatorrhoea (pale stools, characteristically float).
⌘ Constipation with overflow (history of constipation, hard faeces on abdominal or rectal examination, faecal overload on plain abdominal X-ray if still in doubt)
⌘ Rectal discharge.

Step 2. Exclude infection or dehydration

⌘ Modify laxatives if necessary.
⌘ Start loperamide 4 mg single dose, then 2 mg twice a day increasing to 4 mg four times a day according to response.
⌘ Consider pancreatic enzymes if steatorrhoea.
⌘ Consider metronidazole 400 mg three times a day for ten days if bacterial overgrowth likely (blind loop, etc).
⌘ Consider octreotide 300 µg/24 hours. It is parenteral, not all patients respond and it is expensive. Discuss with a specialist team if necessary.

Step 3. Faecal incontinence

Follow steps 1 and 2 above, and see section on incontinence (urinary and faecal, *Section 3.14*) for advice on general care.

3.8 Fatigue

Fatigue is one of the commonest symptoms of advanced cancer (and of many chronic non-cancer illnesses). It is distressing, it impacts significantly on quality of life, and it is often not well addressed.
　It can be divided into:

- **generalized physical weakness**, making it difficult to initiate activities
- **reduced physical stamina**, producing early tiring
- **psychological fatigue** with loss of motivation, drive, memory concentration.

Often patients experience a mixture of all three, which may be further complicated by drowsiness, sleepiness and altered sleep behaviour. A self-sustaining downward spiral can result (see *Figure 3.8.1*).

Causes of fatigue in cancer and chronic illness are almost always complex and multi-factorial. Sometimes it is genuinely not possible to correct, but a systematic approach helps.

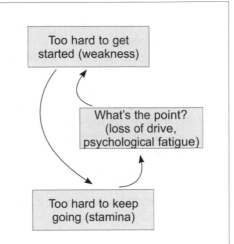

Figure 3.8.1: The fatigue cycle

Step 1. Is there a correctable cause?

⌘ Screen for depression.

⌘ Check for anaemia.

⌘ Check for uraemia, hypercalcaemia, electrolyte disturbances, thyroid function.

⌘ Review drugs, especially sedating drugs (opioids in too big a dose, benzodiazepines) and long-term steroids (steroid-induced proximal myopathy can start after a few weeks of treatment).

⌘ Screen for chronic low-grade infection if suspicion (urine, chest, wound infection).

⌘ Optimize symptom control, especially pain, nausea, vomiting, insomnia.

Step 2. Energy optimization strategy

⌘ Nutritional review with dietary enrichment, food and/or vitamin supplements where indicated.

⌘ Activity planning
- use of pacing (interspersing activity with rest periods)

- practical help with high-energy/low-reward activities, eg. housework, ironing
- regular, gentle exercise
- alter daily time schedule to fit in with daily energy pattern
- arrange for bed/toilet facility easily accessible
- energy conservation techniques (in conjunction with occupational therapist).

⌘ Psychological coping — positive reframing, eg. 'Your body has less energy than usual because it is using its energy to try to fight the cancer' or 'Your body tires more easily because the chemotherapy drugs work like a poison. They are designed to be much more poisonous to the cancer cells than to the rest of your body, but I guess if the rest of your body is noticing the effect, the cancer cells must hopefully be feeling it many times over'.

⌘ Setting realistic goals.

⌘ Maintaining hope.

⌘ Diversional therapy, eg. day hospice.

⌘ Complementary therapies.

Step 3. Prescribing

⌘ Corticosteroids. Dexamethasone 4 mg daily or prednisolone 20–30 mg daily for a one-week trial. If no benefit stop; if helpful, continue on lowest dose that maintains benefit.

⌘ Psychostimulants may be effective. Methylphenidate has been used, particularly where fatigue relates to opioid dose needed for pain control. Discuss with specialist service.

3.9 Fits

Fits are frightening for patient and family. They also impact on the patient's ability to drive, and subsequent independence and quality of life. Wherever possible they should be prevented. Common reasons for fits are failure to anticipate the risk and prescribe prophylactic anticonvulsants, and the sudden withdrawal of anticonvulsants (and/or steroids) as the patient deteriorates and becomes unable to swallow.

Step 1. Prevention

⌘ Anticipate fits in all patients with intracranial malignancy, whether primary or secondary.

⌘ Discuss the use of prophylactic anticonvulsants with colleagues from secondary care (not always indicated).

⌘ Monitor anticonvulsant levels where indicated.

⌘ Anticipate fits when the patient suddenly stops anticonvulsants (eg. as oral intake ceases in the last days of life). Prescribe prophylactic non-oral anticonvulsant, eg. midazolam 30 mg/24 hours subcutaneously via syringe driver, or diazepam rectally. Also prescribe and leave in the house midazolam 10 mg subcutaneous injection or diazepam 10 mg rectally to use in case of fitting.

⌘ Anticipate fits when a patient suddenly stops high-dose steroids prescribed for intracranial malignancy (eg. as oral intake ceases in the last days of life).

⌘ Prescribe prophylactic non-oral anticonvulsant. Midazolam 30 mg/24 hours subcutaneously or diazepam are suitable. Also prescribe and leave in the house midazolam 10 mg subcutaneous injection or diazepam 10 mg rectally to use in case of fitting.

Step 2. Treatment

⌘ Ensure safety.

⌘ Airway.

⌘ Diazepam rectally or midazolam 10 mg subcutaneously, repeated if necessary.

⌘ Start or review anticonvulsant prophylaxis.

⌘ Is admission necessary? (discuss if necessary).

⌘ If staying at home, does the steroid dose need review?

Step 3. Communication and education

⌘ Fits are frightening for patient and family, but can be managed at home.

⌘ Families need to know what to do to assist with overall safety, and care of the airway.

⌘ Families can sometimes administer rectal diazepam or subcutaneous midazolam, but this needs careful negotiation in a frightening situation.

⌘ Families need to know who to call, when and how, eg. dial '999' or telephone the GP surgery.

3.10 Fungating lesions

Any cancer near the skin surface can break down and cause a chronic fungating lesion. This causes major problems for the patient and the family. There is a constant visible reminder of the cancer, and often significant effects on body image, self-esteem and social interaction. There may also be problems with pain, discharge and odour. Management needs the multidisciplinary team.

Can the fungating lesion be controlled by specific therapy?

⌘ Is it secondary to a cancer that may respond to hormone manipulation or chemotherapy? (cancer of the breast for, example.)
⌘ will it respond to radiotherapy?
⌘ Is surgery/wound toilet an option? (occasionally gives good palliation.)

Is the lesion infected?

⌘ Secondary infection is common.
⌘ Swab for bacteriology.
⌘ Oral metronidazole 400 mg three times daily for seven to fourteen days.

Does the lesion smell?

⌘ Secondary anaerobic colonization may produce a foul odour, which is distressing to patient and family.
⌘ Try topical metronidazole gel, either a 200 mg tablet crushed and mixed in 20 g KY jelly or a commercially prepared gel.
⌘ Odour-absorbent dressings. These contain activated charcoal in various arrangements layered with alginate and hydrocolloid where there is heavy exudate, as non-absorbent dressings or layered with polyurethane foam. They are listed under 'Wound management products' in an appendix of the *British National Formulary (BNF)*.

Is there much exudate?

⌘ Most lesions are best cleaned by irrigation with sterile normal saline.

⌘ Alginate, foam, hydrogel and hydrocolloid dressings are all designed to absorb excessive exudate. Alginates and foams can be highly absorbent. Hydrogel dressings are usually more suitable for dry, sloughy or necrotic wounds, and have limited capacity to absorb exudate. Suitable products are listed in the back of the *BNF,* and many areas have nursing protocols.

Is there surface bleeding?

⌘ Consider referral for radiotherapy or laser coagulation.
⌘ Calcium alginate dressings can be haemostatic. Try to reduce dressing frequency to avoid disturbing the bleeding surface.
⌘ Topical sucralfate can be applied as a 1% paste. This is made by crushing 1 g sucralfate and mixing with either 10 g KY jelly or 10 g metronidazole gel (for wounds with co-existing odour).

Is the lesion painful?

⌘ Cutaneous pain does not always respond well to oral strong opioids, but they are worth trying.
⌘ Pain may improve with control of infection.
⌘ Non-steroidal anti-inflammatory drugs may give relief.
⌘ Cutaneous pain may respond to topical morphine. There is currently no commercially available preparation. Centres using topical morphine prepare a 0.1–0.3% gel, which is applied twice-daily.

How does the patient feel?

⌘ Assess mood and coping skills.
⌘ Consider antidepressants, counselling.
⌘ Sustain interest and support.

3.11 Haemorrhage and haemoptysis

General care

⌘ Check clotting and platelets.
⌘ Adjust anticoagulants (consider platelet transfusion if low platelets resulting from chemotherapy), discuss if necessary with haematologist.
⌘ Encourage dark towels/handkerchiefs/underwear if frightened.
⌘ Pads.
⌘ Remember that although major haemorrhage is rare, fear is common (with professionals and patients).
⌘ If major haemorrhage is a risk, assess benefit/risk of preparing patient and/or family and consider making crisis medication easily available (single syringes of diamorphine and midazolam).

Topical treatments

⌘ Alginate dressings, changing as little as possible.
⌘ Topical sucralfate paste (crush 1 g in 10 g water-miscible gel) or 1% alum solution.
⌘ Topical tranexamic acid (soaked onto dressings, as an enema for rectal bleeding or as a mouthwash/gargle for oral bleeding).
⌘ Consider radiotherapy, laser treatment, diathermy.
⌘ Intraluminal treatment may be possible.

Systemic treatments

⌘ Ethamsylate 500 mg four times a day.
⌘ Tranexamic acid 1 g three times a day.

3.12 Hiccoughs

There are many causes, and it is not just as simple as diaphragmatic irritation. It can also be caused by irritation of the vagal or phrenic nerves, uraemia and intracranial pathology. Patients will usually have tried simple non-drug measures. These involve either pharyngeal stimulation (drinking from the wrong side of a cup, swallowing granulated sugar, massaging a cold spoon on the junction of hard and soft palate) or self-induced hypercapnoea (holding the breath or rebreathing into a paper bag). Nebulized saline offers a more 'medical' pharyngeal stimulation.

Step 1. Is this caused by delayed gastric emptying?

⌘ Anti-flatulents (asilone 10–20 ml or Maalox plus) forty-eight-hour trial. If ineffective try metoclopramide 10 mg three times day.
⌘ Stop if not working after forty-eight to seventy-two hours, especially if there is no other evidence of delayed gastric emptying (see nausea and vomiting).

Step 2. Is a diaphragmatic muscle relaxant needed?

⌘ Baclofen 5 mg daily–10 mg twice-daily (higher doses described) *or*
⌘ Nifedipine 10–20 mg three times a day.

Step 3. Is a centrally acting agent needed?

⌘ Consider first with intracranial disease.
⌘ Sodium valproate 200 mg four times a day.
⌘ Chlorpromazine 10–25 mg two to three times a day.
⌘ Haloperidol 1.5–3 mg once daily.

Many other interventions are described, possibly more than for most symptoms, which may be indicative of the lack of one simple and reliable intervention.

3.13 Hypercalcaemia

What is hypercalcaemia?

Hypercalcaemia is a raised level of *corrected* calcium in the blood (*total* plasma calcium is the combination of free, ionized calcium and protein-bound calcium. If the albumin level is low, protein-bound calcium is low. This may mask a high concentration of free, ionized calcium. Calcium is 'corrected' for albumin level).

Why is it important?

1. It may cause symptoms. These do not always relate to the level of serum calcium. Common symptoms are:
   * polyuria, polydipsia
   * vomiting
   * constipation
   * tiredness and lethargy
   * muscle weakness
   * confusion
   * coma.
2. It may cause pain, or make existing pain worse.
3. It may cause dehydration, coma and cardiac arrest.

How common is it?

⌘ 10–20% of all patients with cancer.
⌘ 20–40% of patients with cancer of the bronchus, breast or myeloma will have hypercalcaemia.

What sort of cancer produces hypercalcaemia?

⌘ Myeloma is the most likely tumour to produce hypercalcaemia (one-third of patients admitted to hospital).

⌘ Carcinoma of lung and breast account for over half the cases seen.
⌘ Carcinoma of stomach and large bowel rarely produce hypercalcaemia.

Hypercalcaemia of malignancy is caused by the secretion of a parathyroid hormone-like substance by the tumour. Contrary to popular belief, it can occur in the absence of bone metastases. Conversely, patients can have widespread bone metastases and remain normocalcaemic.

What is the significance of hypercalcaemia?

Hypercalcaemia usually indicates disseminated disease (74%). Ninety-five percent of patients with breast cancer and hypercalcaemia have disseminated disease; 61% of patients with lung cancer and hypercalcaemia have disseminated disease.

There are only *four* cases in the world literature of a cure in the presence of malignant hypercalcaemia; hypercalcaemia usually means a poor prognosis — four-fifths of patients die within a year.

Treatment

Treatment is aimed at improving wellbeing and symptoms for symptomatic patients for weeks or even months. The treatment of choice is an intravenous bisphosphonate infusion (pamidronate). Zoledronic acid is even more potent. Before treatment, the following need to be considered:

• is the patient symptomatic or is the serum corrected calcium >3 mmol/l?
• is this the first episode? If so, an oncology opinion is warranted. A change in anti-tumour therapy may be indicated
• is the patient's quality of life good (in his or her opinion)?
• is the patient willing to undergo intravenous therapy/blood tests?
• will the treatment work? (what response was there to previous treatment?)

Treatment is usually simple and well tolerated. Sometimes transient flu-like symptoms occur, which respond to oral paracetamol. A typical dosing schedule for pamidronate is given in *Table 3.13.1*.

The dose is made up in 500 ml of N-saline and given over two hours. With appropriate supervision and training it can be given in day-case units, community hospitals or in the home if nursing support is available.

It takes up to three days to start working, and five to seven days to exert its maximum effect. Patients who are symptomatic, clinically dehydrated or with a calcium >3.5 will need admitting for rehydration for three days while it takes effect. The dose can be repeated after a week if the initial response is inadequate.

Zoledronic acid 4 mg is as effective as pamidronate 90 mg, can be given intravenously over five to ten minutes and response can last up to five weeks. This makes it advantageous in a primary-care setting, but choice of bisphosphonate may depend on local guidelines and protocols.

Table 3.13.1: Typical dosing schedule for pamidronate

Corrected serum calcium (mmol/l)	Pamidronate dose (mg)
3	15–30
3–3.5	30–60
3.5–4	60–90
>4	90

How long does treatment last?

A single infusion will usually maintain normocalcaemia for three weeks. Hypercalcaemia tends to recur. Consider monitoring the serum calcium weekly and ensure the patient and family know the symptoms to watch for. Pamidronate infusions can be repeated every three to four weeks according to the serum calcium. There is no evidence that oral bisphosphonates prevent further episodes of hypercalcaemia, and they are poorly tolerated.

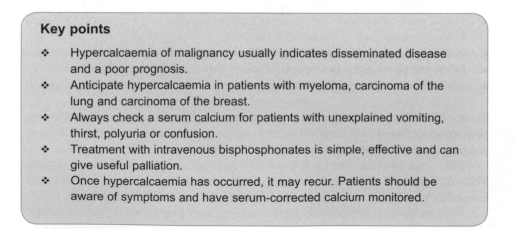

Key points

❖ Hypercalcaemia of malignancy usually indicates disseminated disease and a poor prognosis.

❖ Anticipate hypercalcaemia in patients with myeloma, carcinoma of the lung and carcinoma of the breast.

❖ Always check a serum calcium for patients with unexplained vomiting, thirst, polyuria or confusion.

❖ Treatment with intravenous bisphosphonates is simple, effective and can give useful palliation.

❖ Once hypercalcaemia has occurred, it may recur. Patients should be aware of symptoms and have serum-corrected calcium monitored.

3.14 Incontinence (urinary and faecal)

Urinary incontinence is generally manageable. Faecal incontinence is difficult and a common cause of total care breakdown. Urinary or faecal incontinence engender feelings of childlikeness, of loss of control and dignity, and can impact on carers as much as patients. Practical aspects such as managing odour, laundry and skin care are often basic concerns (*Table 3.14.1*).

Table 3.14.1: Practical care for urinary and faecal incontinence	
Odour	Hygiene Regular clothes changes/laundry Deodorizing spray, essential oils, environmental air filters
Laundry	Protective covers for chairs/bedding Pads/containment garments Local services where available Liaise with social services
Skincare	Cleanliness/drying Dimeticone-based creams (Siopel or Conotrane) Zinc-based creams (zinc and castor oil) Treat thrush/dermatitis

Urinary incontinence

Step 1. Is this caused by retention/overflow?

* Bladder palpable abdominally.
* Catheterize.
* Treat cause if possible.

Step 2. Is this caused by a fistula?

* Clinical picture is of constant, low-volume dribbling day and night.
* Urinary leakage PV, PR or through perineal skin.
* Urine may contain faecal matter/frequent infections.

⌘ If doubt, methylene blue can be instilled into bladder (liaise with urologist).

Management: urinary fistula

- plan regular (hourly) micturition with pads/skincare
- trial of catheterization (does not always help)
- vaginal tampons may control vaginal leak in vesico-vaginal fistula
- liaise with specialist services (depending on patient's overall level of fitness).

Step 3. Is it worth a trial of medication?

Sometimes helpful for unstable bladder:

- oxybutinin 2.5–5 mg twice to four times a day (or modified-release formulation)
- tolterodine 2 mg twice a day
- imipramine 10–50 mg at night
- propantheline 15–30 mg three times a day
- if nocturnal incontinence disturbs sleep, try desmopressin 200–400µg orally or 20–40 µg intranasal spray once-daily at bedtime. (The patient should avoid fluid overload for eight hours after the spray, and plasma sodium should be monitored — get advice on this first.)

Step 4. Containment

Sometimes none of the above work or are appropriate, and the situation needs to be managed and contained:

- liaise with nurse advisor where possible
- pads/pants
- sheaths for men
- intermittent self-catheterization
- indwelling catheter.

Faecal incontinence

⌘ General care as above.
⌘ Refer to section on diarrhoea *(Section 3.7, p. 58)*: is there a treatable cause.
⌘ Consider actively managed bowel movements. Modify laxative/anti-diarrhoeal drugs so the patient is mildly constipated. Every one to three days, depending on degree of control, give a micro-enema or a glycerine plus bisacodyl suppository with ready access to toilet/commode or pad if bedbound.
⌘ Maximize carer support.

3.15 Itching

Causes of itching

⌘ Para-neoplastic.
⌘ Iron deficiency.
⌘ Metabolic, eg. uraemia, raised bilirubin.
⌘ Drug-induced.
⌘ Skin problems, eg. eczema, itch around pressure areas; do not forget common problems such as fungal infection and scabies.

Management of itching

⌘ Simple interventions, avoiding obvious precipitants such as rough or synthetic clothing, or too much heat.
⌘ Try simple emollients. Aqueous cream with or without 5% menthol is soothing. A 5% vinegar solution has also been described as soothing.
⌘ Sedative antihistamines such as chlorpheniramine (chlorphenamine) 4 mg three times a day or promethazine 25 mg at night may help, although one study showed nitrazepam to be just as effective.
⌘ Adding in H_2-receptor blockade with cimetidine 400 mg twice-daily sometimes helps.
⌘ Paroxetine 10 mg daily has been used with benefit for paraneoplastic itch.
⌘ Itching secondary to cholestatic jaundice may improve with stanozolol 5 mg daily (discontinued 2002 — danazol may have similar role, but no UK licence yet).

3.16 Lymphoedema and oedema

> Not all oedema is lymphoedema.

Lymphoedema is only one cause of a swollen limb. Other causes are also common. It helps to be able to differentiate lymphoedema from other swollen limbs for treatment planning. Lymphoedema treatment in particular needs commitment from the patient and healthcare team. It needs to be sustained to remain effective.

Normally, the flow of fluid into soft tissues via capillary filtration equals the flow of fluid out of the soft tissues via the lymphatic drainage system.

> In a normal limb, capillary filtration = lymphatic drainage.

Limbs swell when capillary filtration (flow of fluid out of the capillaries into soft tissue) exceeds lymphatic drainage. This is simple plumbing. The commonest reason for this is raised capillary filtration. This decompensates lymphatic drainage (even quicker if the latter is impaired), which causes **water** to accumulate in the limb and produces **oedema** (*Figure 3.16.1*).

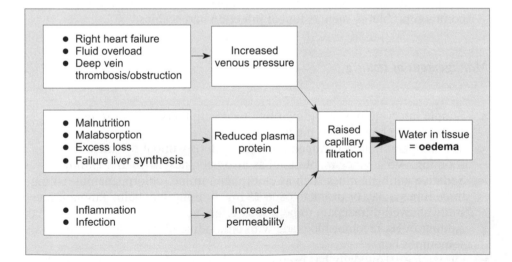

Figure 3.16.1: Causes of oedema

Oedema may be secondary to a mixture of these different causes. For example, legs mildly swollen by heart failure may become much more swollen if an episode of cellulitis intervenes. Infections can cause swollen limbs to deteriorate in two ways: not only do they increase capillary permeability and leakage of fluid into the limb; they can also damage lymphatic drainage.

What is lymphoedema?

If lymphatic drainage is insufficient, lymph accumulates in the soft tissue of the limb. Lymph consists not only of water, but also of protein, fat, cells and so on. The accumulation of this fluid is lymphoedema. It can be primary or secondary.

Why do lymphatics fail?

The lymphatics are a fine network of drainage channels that lead into drainage lymphatics. These drain the limb, eventually re-joining the systemic circulation via the thoracic duct. Lymphatic insufficiency arises because:

⌘ There are too few lymphatics in the first place:
  • congenital lymphoedema (ask about family history)
  • acquired either from clotting or inflammation (lymphangitis or cellulitis). Ask about deep vein thrombosis/infection.
⌘ The pump in the drainage lymphatics fails.
⌘ The lymphatics are normal, but the flow is obstructed, eg. by surgery (block dissections), lymphatic infiltration or scarring (including post-radiotherapy).
⌘ The system is overloaded, leading to incompetence and reflux.

Clinical situations with a high risk of lymphoedema

⌘ Breast cancer after radiotherapy or axillary node dissection.
⌘ Radiotherapy to the axilla, inguinal or pelvic areas.
⌘ Block dissection of axillary, inguinal or pelvic nodes.
⌘ Advanced cancers with massive lymphatic involvement.

Step 1. Is this lymphoedema? (see Table 3.16.1)

The clinical changes visible in the limb are a consequence of the presence of the rich, high-protein lymphatic fluid in the subcutaneous tissue. This produces (according to severity and duration):

- cool, pale skin
- increased limb volume
- thickened skin, fibrosis, possibly pitting
- thickened skin folds, hyperkeratosis, verrucous projections if longstanding
- lymphorrhoea if severe
- like oedema, may involve the truncal quadrant
- typically does not respond to elevation (but reduces lymph flow, which may give comfort)
- typically does not improve overnight.

Table 3.16.1: Distinguishing lymphoedema from other causes of oedema

Diagnosis	Key clinical clues
Heart failure	Pitting oedema, improves with elevation/overnight Check for cardiomegaly/raised jugular venous pressure
Venous obstruction	Venous dilatation May be dusky discoloration
Inferior vena cava obstruction	Massive bilateral and genital oedema
Venous hypertension	Reddish discoloration (red blood cells forced out) Varicosities Venous ulceration
Low albumin	Massive bilateral/genital oedema May become more generalized Check plasma proteins

Step 2. If this is lymphoedema, is the patient suitable for treatment?

⌘ *Is the patient motivated?*
Lymphoedema treatment is hard work. It controls rather than cures, so is life-long. The patient needs to be sufficiently troubled by the symptom to want to engage in treatment

⌘ *Is treatment likely to be worthwhile?*
- is the patient physically fit enough to comply?
- is the family/district nursing support adequate?
- is the benefit worth the effort?

- sometimes if a patient has multiple pathologies, is relatively immobile or wheelchair bound and the swollen limbs are asymptomatic, treatment can be an unnecessary burden.
⌘ *Is treatment safe?*
  - is it likely to precipitate fluid overload/heart failure?
  - is the arterial circulation adequate?
⌘ *Is there undiagnosed recurrence?*
  - look for abdominal/pelvic pathology
  - check axillary/groin glands
  - discuss with diagnostic consultant/oncologist if doubt.

Step 3. Treat (Table 3.16.2)

⌘ Only lymphoedema benefits from lymphoedema treatment.
⌘ Look at the whole patient.
⌘ Mixed pathology may need multiple interventions.
⌘ Always look for and treat aggressively tinea pedis, bacterial infection (penicillin V 250 mg four times a day for fourteen days), dermatitis.
⌘ Contain lymphorrhea with pads/bandages awaiting any specialist assessment.
⌘ Refer if possible to a specialist lymphoedema clinic, which can assess, measure, monitor and provide a range of interventions.

Key points

- ❖ Not all swollen limbs are caused by lymphoedema.
- ❖ Most forms of oedema respond to low-pressure stockings (class 1 or 2) and treatment of the cause.
- ❖ Lymphoedema produces a recognizable clinical picture with typically non-gravity-dependant oedema.
- ❖ Treatment requires commitment from patient and staff; it is life-long.
- ❖ Referral to a specialist lymphoedema service is helpful.

Table 3.16.2: Treatment for lymphoedema and other causes of oedema

Cause of limb swelling	Treatments to consider
Core lymphoedema treatment	**Skin care** • Regular moisturising with simple emollients • Chiropody/care with fingernails • Fast-track access to antibiotics at first sign of infection; consider leaving patient with a supply to start if needed • Avoid injury (including injection/intravenous cannulation) to the affected limb **Exercise** **Truncal massage** • Various techniques • Family member may help • Circular motion with fingers or electric massager **Support/compression** • TED stockings are not appropriate — compression garments for lymphoedema are different and need fitting professionally • Need to be worn before starting to use the limb • In an ill patient who is too unwell to attend clinic, it may be worth a trial of spironolactone 100–200 mg daily with bandaging for comfort
Heart failure	Diuretics Low-pressure stockings (class 1 or 2)
Venous obstruction	?Anticoagulants Stents Steroids (dexamethasone 8 mg once daily for a week) Anti-tumour treatment Low-pressure stockings (class 1 or 2) Half-leg bandaging/truncal massage if severe
Low albumin	High protein diet Whole blood transfusion? Low-pressure stockings (class 1 or 2) Half-leg bandaging/truncal massage if severe

3.17 Mouth care

> *Everything is relative. A sore mouth does not suggest agony beyond endurance. I felt embarrassed by it. I was really embarrassed by my pain, embarrassed by my inability to eat.* **Cancer patient with mucositis**

Disorders or discomfort of the mouth can seem comparatively trivial to both patients and healthcare workers, compared with the main disease process.

However, the mouth is a vital organ and is essential for core daily activities such as eating, drinking and communicating. Dysfunction or pain can cause much distress. Patients should be routinely offered basic advice about mouthcare. Common problems are:

- thrush
- mouth ulcers
- oral pain
- excessive salivation and drooling.

> Basic mouth care = keep the mouth moist and keep the mouth clean

Keeping the mouth moist

A dry mouth is common, is exacerbated by many medications and predisposes to soreness. Try:

- frequent sips or sprays of plain or mineral water
- sucking pineapple chunks (tinned can be kept in the fridge and easily accessed; fresh works better), ice cubes, frozen fruit juice
- refreshing mouthwashes, eg. 50% cider/50% soda water or effervescent mouthwash tablets
- chewing gum
- sucking fruit sweets.

Consider prescribing:

- saliva-stimulating tablets (SST)
- artificial saliva sprays, lozenges or gels
- pilocarpine tablets 5–10 mg three times a day.

Keeping the mouth clean

- tooth-brushing twice a day
- one-quarter of a 1 g effervescent ascorbic acid tablet dissolved on the tongue
- antiseptic mouthwashes sparingly.

Thrush

Diagnose by:

- white patches on mucosa and/or
- atrophic glossitis (smooth red tongue) and/or
- angular cheilitis (cracks in corners of mouth)
- mouth swabs not usually useful (positive in 40–60% of a normal, asymptomatic population).

Treat with:

- fluconazole 50 mg once a day for seven days
- fluconazole 150 mg single dose
- nystatin 2 ml four times a day. Often ineffective; difficult to use. Note 1 ml four times a day insufficient
- ketoconazole 200 mg once a day for five days
- sterilize dentures.

Mouth ulcers

Treat with:

- choline salicylate gel (Bonjela®)
- topical steroid, eg. triamcinolone (Adcortyl®) in orabase
- tetracycline mouthwash, 250 mg capsule opened into water, then held in the mouth for two minutes three times a day
- for malignant ulcers with secondary infection, consider a course of metronidazole or flucloxacillin orally.

Oral pain

Treat the cause plus:

- benzydamine spray or mouthwash (Difflam®)
- choline salicylate gel (Bonjela®)
- sucralfate suspension 10 ml four times a day (mucosal protectant — use as a mouthwash and hold in the mouth for several minutes)
- topical non-steroidal anti-inflammatory drugs
- systemic analgesia.

Excessive salivation and drooling

Try:

- hyoscine hydrobromide sublingually or transdermally (1 mg/72 hours)
- atropine 0.4 mg four times a day orally (rarely used)
- beta-blockers, eg. propanolol 10 mg twice a day or metoprolol 25 mg twice a day (especially for motor neurone disease [MND] patients with thick secretions)
- propantheline.

3.18 Nausea and vomiting

Good management of nausea and vomiting is one of the biggest therapeutic challenges in palliative care. Nineteen different anti-emetics are listed in the *BNF*. This does not include a separate listing for prokinetic agents. Despite this, many of us were brought up on domperidone, metoclopramide and prochlorperazine, and when these are ineffective we are left adrift. Good management of nausea and vomiting means knowing or making an educated guess at the likeliest cause. This enables us to choose the drug most likely to be effective scientifically, based on the underlying physiology (*Table 3.18.1*).

This need not be complex; using just three drugs well and appropriately gives a strong framework from which to start.

Step 1. Think of correctable causes

⌘ Check the calcium and urea.
⌘ Check for gaseous distension, high-pitched bowel sounds and colic (could this be a correctable bowel obstruction?)
⌘ Ask about headache, visual disturbance and check the fundi if indicated (could this be raised intracranial pressure? Rare without concomitant headache).

Discuss management of correctable causes with your specialist palliative care team.

Table 3.18.1. Cause and treatment of nausea and vomiting

Commonest causes	Physiological site	Best drug acting at that site
Radiotherapy Anxiety Vagally mediated: gastrointestinal distension (eg. obstruction/ genitourinary distension)	Vomiting centre	**Cyclizine** 25–50 mg three times a day orally, subcutaneously or rectally
Drugs (eg. opiates) Metabolic (raised Ca^{2+} urea) Toxins (eg. tumour toxins)	CTZ*	**Haloperidol** 1.5 mg daily, orally or subcutaneously
Drugs (particularly those with anticholinergic side effects) Outflow obstruction (tumour or hepatomegaly) Squashed stomach (tumour, ascites)	Gastric stasis	**Metoclopramide** 30–60 mg orally or subcutaneously, or domperidone 30–60 mg rectally every 8 hours

*CTZ = chemoreceptor trigger zone in the floor of the fourth ventricle of the brain

Step 2. Is a prokinetic drug (ie. metoclopramide) indicated?

⌘ Prokinetics promote gastric emptying.

⌘ They are the drug of choice for delayed gastric emptying or gastric stasis.

⌘ This gives a typical vomiting pattern of large-volume vomits, often worse later in the day, which may contain food eaten several hours previously. Heartburn, hiccoughs and early satiation confirm the clinical diagnosis. Nausea is not a major feature and is relieved by vomiting

⌘ If you elicit this vomiting pattern, prescribe metoclopramide 10–20 mg three times a day orally half an hour before meals

⌘ If the patient is vomiting more than two to three times a day, or the vomiting does not settle within two to three days of oral medication, prescribe metoclopramide 30–60 mg over twenty-four hours by syringe driver.

Step 3. Is the vomiting caused by opioids or a chemical/metabolic cause?

⌘ Opioid-induced vomiting is diagnosed by a careful vomiting history confirming a clear relationship between starting the opioid and the onset of vomiting (within the first hours/days).

⌘ If a patient has been on opioids for some time and starts vomiting, another cause is likely (even if there has been a recent dose change).

⌘ Haloperidol 1.5–3 mg as a single, daily dose is the anti-emetic of choice for opioid-induced vomiting; it acts directly on the chemoreceptor trigger zone.

⌘ Most patients develop tolerance to opioid-induced vomiting over a couple of weeks, allowing the haloperidol to be discontinued.

⌘ A small proportion of patients on opioids also develop a secondary gastric stasis. If haloperidol alone does not settle the vomiting, add in metoclopramide 10 mg three times a day.

⌘ If opioid-induced vomiting still persists, an alternative strong opioid is indicated.

⌘ For chemical and metabolic causes, such as hypercalcaemia and uraemia, start with haloperidol again at 1.5–3 mg as a single, daily dose.

Step 4. Is the patient still vomiting?

⌘ Have you followed steps 1, 2 and 3? Have you corrected any underlying cause?

⌘ Is the patient complying with medication and is it being absorbed?

⌘ If the patient is vomiting more than two to three times a day, oral anti-emetics are unlikely to be effective as they are unlikely to be absorbed.

⌘ A syringe driver bypasses the oral route and will ensure a fair trial of the anti-emetic.

⌘ Explain this to the patient and prescribe the same medication via syringe driver, at least until the vomiting is controlled.

⌘ Consider cyclizine 25–50 mg orally three times a day, or 75–150 mg via a syringe driver. It is effective for a range of causes of vomiting, although it is sometimes poorly tolerated because of dryness of the mouth, drowsiness or skin irritation from subcutaneous use.

⌘ Cyclizine and haloperidol are a potent combination well worth trying.

⌘ Do not combine cyclizine with metoclopramide; they oppose each others' action.

⌘ Levomepromazine (Nozinan®) 3–25 mg daily orally or subcutaneously is a broad-spectrum anti-emetic. It can be given at higher doses (up to 100–150 mg a day) for vomiting with agitation, but is sedating at these doses.

Step 5. If all else fails

⌘ Get specialist help if available.

⌘ Levomepromazine (Nozinan®) 3–25 mg orally or 6.25–25 mg subcutaneously (can be given as a single, daily dose at night). Acts on multiple receptor sites, but can cause unacceptable sedation in the ambulant patient. Can be used in doses up to 150 mg daily in patients with agitation and vomiting and/or in end-of-life care.

⌘ Octreotide (usually with specialist supervision/advice).

⌘ Dexamethasone 8 mg daily has anti-emetic activity.

⌘ Consider a nasogastric tube (or venting gastrosomy).

See *Table 3.18.2. (opposite)* for nausea and vomiting protocol.

3.19 Spinal cord compression

What is malignant spinal cord compression?

A real emergency

Tumour (usually a bony metastasis in the vertebra) grows and presses on the spinal cord. Initially, there may be pain and tenderness at the site of the metastasis. Ninety-five percent of patients give a history of back pain in the preceding six to seven weeks. As the tumour grows, increasing pressure on the spinal cord reaches a critical point and often suddenly produces:

• weakness (usually bilateral)
• sensory disturbance (late sign)
• sphincter disturbance (late sign).

If undetected or untreated this can rapidly progress to:

• paralysis (very late sign)
• numbness (very late sign)
• double incontinence (very late sign).

Table 3.18.2: Protocol for nausea and vomiting

- Assess cause — start a vomiting diary
- If vomiting is once a day or more, give anti-emetics parenterally initially

Cause	Site	Step 1	Step 2 (if partial/no response to step 1)	Step 3 (if partial/no response to step 2)	If all else fails
DXR + raised intracranial pressure Anxiety Vagus-gastrointestinal or urinary tract distension (including constipation, bowel obstruction)	Vomiting centre	Cyclizine 25–50 mg three times a day, orally, subcutaneously, or rectally	Add haloperidol 1.5–10 mg once a day orally or subcutaneously	Intestinal obstruction – add octreotide 300 µg – 600 µg/24 hours	Get specialist help
Chemotherapy Drugs (opiates) Metabolic (calcium, urea) Toxins (including tumour load)	*CTZ	Haloperidol 1.5–10 mg daily, orally or subcutaneously	Chemotherapy – substitute ondansetron Metabolic – add cyclizine Opiate-induced – add metoclopramide	Anxiety/chemotherapy – add lorazepam or	Consider either Dexamethasone 8 mg once a day
Drugs (anticholinergic) Outflow obstruction Squashed stomach (hepatomegaly, large tumour mass)	Gastric stasis	Metoclopramide 30–60 mg orally or subcutaneously or Domperidone 30–60 mg rectally 8-hourly		? Nasogastric tube	Levomepromazine (Nozinan) 12.5 mg once daily

At each step:
- Reassess cause
- Stop all anti-emetics that are not working
- Avoid combinations of more than two anti-emetics if possible
- Reassess carefully and see if simpler and more specific treatment is possible

*CTZ=chemoreceptor trigger zone in the floor of the fourth ventricle of the brain

Why is it important?

Early detection and treatment can **prevent** paralysis and double incontinence. It is not a fatal condition, and 30% of patients will survive at least a year. Although rare, it is devastating if diagnosed too late as irreversible paraplegia ensues:

- 70% of patients walking at the time of diagnosis retain their mobility
- <5% of patients with paraplegia at the time of diagnosis regain any mobility.

How common is it?

Cord compression affects 5% of all cancer patients. Cancer of the breast, lung and prostate account for two-thirds of cases.

Symptoms (Figure 3.19.1)

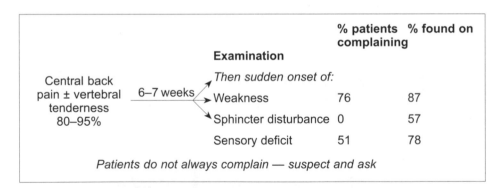

			% patients complaining	% found on
		Examination		
Central back pain ± vertebral tenderness 80–95%	6–7 weeks	*Then sudden onset of:*		
		Weakness	76	87
		Sphincter disturbance	0	57
		Sensory deficit	51	78

Patients do not always complain — suspect and ask

Figure 3.19.1: Symptoms of spinal cord compression (Kramer, 1992)

What sort of pain occurs in spinal cord compression?

- Local bone pain in the back, particularly the **thoracic spine (80%)**, often worse lying down and better sitting up.
- Nerve root compression pain (radicular pain). Can be unilateral or bilateral, sharp, may be jabbing or stabbing.

⌘ Cord compression pain (funicular pain) goes around the limb in a 'cuff' or 'garter' pattern, often knees, calves or thighs. Diffuse, cold, unpleasant sensation.

Both radicular and funicular pain is made worse by:

- flexing the neck
- straight leg raising
- coughing, sneezing or straining.

> This is the stage to suspect and diagnose.

Once weakness, sphincter disturbance and sensory deficit have arisen, they progress rapidly. The likelihood of a good outcome from treatment falls rapidly.

What sort of tests?

⌘ Plain X-ray of the spine is quick and has diagnostic accuracy of 80% (60% for bone scan). X-ray cervical, thoracic, lumbar spine and pelvis
⌘ Magnetic resonance imaging (MRI) scan (urgently within twenty-four hours) is the imaging modality of choice.
⌘ A normal plain x-ray and bone scan do NOT exclude malignant cord compression.

Treatment

Treatment is *always* indicated, unless the patient is moribund (*Figure 3.19.2*). Functional outcome is listed in *Table 3.19.2*.

Table 3.19.2: Functional outcome after treatment of spinal cord compression	
Mobility at presentation	**% Mobile after treatment***
Ambulant	50–80%
Paretic	30–40%
Paraplegic	5%
*25% relapse within 6 months	

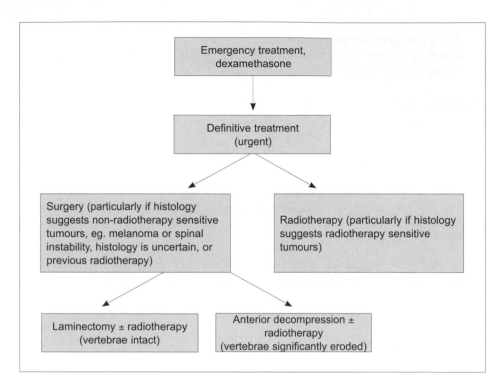

Figure 3.19.2: Treatment of spinal cord compression

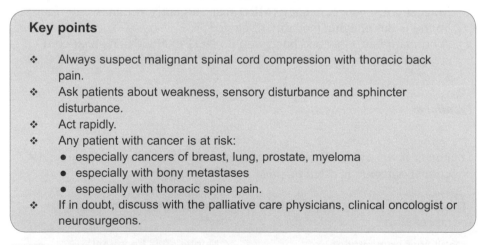

Key points

❖ Always suspect malignant spinal cord compression with thoracic back pain.

❖ Ask patients about weakness, sensory disturbance and sphincter disturbance.

❖ Act rapidly.

❖ Any patient with cancer is at risk:
- especially cancers of breast, lung, prostate, myeloma
- especially with bony metastases
- especially with thoracic spine pain.

❖ If in doubt, discuss with the palliative care physicians, clinical oncologist or neurosurgeons.

Bibliography

Husband DJ (1998) Malignant spinal cord compression; prospective study of delays in referral and treatment. *Br Med J* **317**: 18–22

Kramer JA (1992) *Palliative Medicine* **6**: 202–11

3.20 Sweating

Common causes

- ⌘ Infection.
- ⌘ Paraneoplastic sweating.
- ⌘ Hormonal.

Management

- ⌘ Simple measures, avoiding excessive heat, maintaining fluid intake, light clothing.
- ⌘ Exclude or treat infection.
- ⌘ Paracetamol 1 g four times a day.
- ⌘ Non-steroidal anti-inflammatory drugs, eg. naproxen 500 mg twice a day.
- ⌘ Corticosteroids, eg. dexamethasone 4 mg once a day.
- ⌘ Propranolol.
- ⌘ Propantheline 15–30 mg two to three times a day.
- ⌘ Amitriptyline 10–50 mg at night.

For hormonal sweating consider

- ⌘ Hormone replacement therapy if no contraindication.
- ⌘ Medroxyprogesterone acetate 5–20 mg twice a day or megestrol acetate.
- ⌘ 40 mg once a day (takes two to four weeks to work).
- ⌘ Venlafaxine 37.5 mg twice a day.
- ⌘ Clonidine 100 μg once a day.

3.21 Terminal restlessness and agitation

As death approaches, between 40–80% of patients may experience motor restlessness, fear, anxiety, mental confusion with or without hallucinations, or a combination of these symptoms (see *Figure 3.21.1*).

In this situation:

⌘ Check for basic comfort, eg. smooth bedclothes, ensure patient not too tightly tucked in, prevent excessive heat/cold.
⌘ Exclude a full bladder or rectum.
⌘ Is the patient in pain?
⌘ Is there a need to have a family member visit or reconciliation/ forgiveness/permission to move on? Even if the patient appears unconscious, he or she may respond to words spoken by a significant person (see also *Chapter 22*).
⌘ Sedation may be necessary. Always explain what you are offering to the patient if possible, and to the family; 'We can make you more comfortable and less frightened, but this may mean you are more sleepy; is that OK?'
⌘ Haloperidol 5–10 mg/24 hours subcutaneously will usually settle confusion/hallucinations (occasionally higher doses are necessary).
⌘ Midazolam 10–30 mg/24 hours subcutaneously will usually provide relief of motor restlessness, fear and useful sedation (occasionally higher doses are necessary).

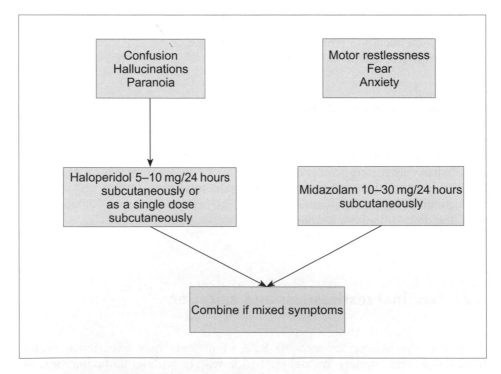

Figure 3.21.1: Terminal restlessness and agitation

4

Nutrition and nourishment

This section deals with issues connected with nutrition that are commonly brought to the primary healthcare team. Nutrition is a core human concern and activity. Much of this section will focus on more technical aspects of dietary components and how to help patients optimize their nutritional intake.

The patient and family are starting from a different place. Food is nourishment. It represents nurturing. The preparing and sharing of food is an activity whereby human beings show love and caring for each other. It builds and maintains relationships, and permeates most aspects of social function. Much of popular culture is concerned with food, recipes, celebrity chefs and diets. Mealtimes come round with great regularity. Most rituals and celebrations in most cultures involve the preparation and sharing of food. In illness, food preparation is often even more ritualized, and careful preparation of foods perceived as nourishing are widely regarded as a key part of the invalid's recovery programme.

Against this background it is not difficult to see the sense of loss, distress and fear that an inability to eat 'normally' can engender. The loss of weight and physical weakness are visible reminders of the continuing presence of serious illness. The loss of the ability to enjoy favourite foods and drinks is a real loss for many patients. The constant careful preparation of foods once enjoyed, but now rejected, can be wearing to the morale of the carer. Any intervention to help nutritional intake needs to engage the carers as much as the patient, with shared, achievable and appropriate goals. It will need to be well negotiated and will work best if it incorporates as much as possible of familiar and favourite foods.

The patient with normal appetite

4.1 Advising on the role of nutrition in the treatment of cancer

There is a considerable body of literature on the role of nutrition in the prevention of cancer. A comprehensive review by Sandra Goodman refers to some 5000 published studies by 1993! The main dietary recommendations are to introduce substantial and varied amounts of fruit and vegetables into the diet and to keep alcohol intake within recommended limits. Other recommendations are to reduce the amount of red meat and processed meats in the diet, to increase the amount of dietary fibre and to maintain a healthy body weight (body mass index 20–25). Pulses and whole grains may also offer some protection against cancer.

There is rather less evidence about the role of dietary modification once cancer is present. Many patients may wish to try, and this gives a sense of control back to the patient in a situation in which he or she may otherwise feel powerless. The broad guidelines above, which are known to prevent cancer, are unlikely to cause harm, and by optimizing intake of basic nutrients, vitamins, minerals and anti-oxidants may help to support the body's own healing mechanisms.

4.2 Extreme diets

Sometimes patients ask about more extreme dietary therapies. Examples are the Gerson diet, the raw food diet, the energy diet and the macrobiotic diet. These diets may be diametrically opposed to each other in basic principles and philosophy. They may claim to cure cancer. Some individuals can respond well to such interventions and there are anecdotal case reports of remission or even cure. For most cancer patients, however, these diets are:

- too high in bulk
- too low in calories
- too low in protein
- too tiring and complex to adhere to
- too expensive.

These diets can be a problem if the patient is experiencing reduced appetite and early satiation as a direct tumour effect, and can result in weight loss and a more rapid deterioration.

4.3 The Bristol diet

The Bristol Cancer Help Centre popularized dietary interventions for patients with cancer, thus patients refer to the 'Bristol diet'. This is not a strict diet, but dietary guidelines (*Table 4.3.1*).

Table 4.3.1: 'Bristol diet' guidelines*

Avoid or minimize	Tobacco, alcohol Tea, coffee, caffeine drinks Excessive salt, chemical preservatives, processed foods Sugar Saturated fat, hydrogenated margarine Deep-fried foods Red meat, smoked and cured meat
Eat in moderation	Eggs, dairy produce Fish, preferably deep-sea oily fish (salmon, tuna, mackerel, herring, pilchards pilchards) White meat and poultry (preferably organic)
Eat liberally	Whole grains (brown rice, barley, oats, millet, rye, wheat, corn) Vegetables and fruits Legumes (peas, beans, legumes, sprouted seeds) Seeds (sesame, sunflower, pumpkin) Nuts Water (filtered)

*Based on Goodman *et al* (1994) and Goodman (2001)

4.4 The role of vitamins and supplements

Overall there is modest evidence that vitamins and supplements may have a role in preventing some cancers. Extrapolating from this and from *in-vitro* studies, some patients use nutritional supplements or high-dose vitamins in the hope they will maintain remission and prevent recurrent disease. A small American study (Jatoi *et al*, 1998) evaluated survival in a group of 36 postoperative patients with non-small-cell lung cancer. They found those who took vitamin supplements were more likely to be long-term survivors (41 months *vs* 11 months; *P*=0.002).

The patient with reduced appetite and weight loss

Most patients with cancer will experience eating problems and weight loss at some stage of their illness. Loss of appetite and weight loss is associated with a poor prognosis: they also affect mood, body image, and sense of well being and quality of life. For many patients, discussion and setting realistic eating goals, with consideration of the use of a corticosteroid or a progestogen (see anorexia/cachexia) will bring sufficient benefit.

4.5 Nutritional support for the patient with reduced appetite (see also section on anorexia for pharmacological approaches [*Section 3.1, p. 46*])

Nutritional supplementation is useful for subgroups of patients:

- peri-operatively
- severely malnourished patients
- bone marrow transplant patients
- head and neck cancer patients.

In patients without cancer, malnutrition can lead to impaired T-cell, humoral and mucosal immunity, and malnourished patients are more prone to infection. However, in patients with cancer, the situation is not as clear cut. The role of nutritional supplementation for most patients with cancer is not well established. Cancer-related cachexia syndrome is complex. As well as reduced calorie intake, these patients have raised resting energy expenditure and evidence of a cytokine-mediated generalized inflammatory response. Increasing protein and/ or calorie intake in these patients does not appear to produce benefit.

Not all commercially available supplements are palatable. Many doctors and nurses will have the experience of finding cupboards full of unopened cartons in the patient's home. A supplement-tasting session at a practice meeting will quickly establish why this happens so often, and also the enormous variation in taste and texture between different brands. Despite this, many patients and families value feeling they have tried to improve their nutritional intake. The simplest and most palatable way to do this is by dietary enrichment. The ideas below can be put into a simple leaflet for patients, or your local hospital or community dietician may have one the practice can use.

Adding extra energy and protein to ordinary foods

❖ **Fortified milk** — made by putting two tablespoons of dried milk powder into a pint of full-cream milk. It can be used in drinks and for cooking in place of ordinary milk. It can be used on cereal or to make up deserts, milk puddings or soups.

❖ **Butter/margarine.** Can be used to add calories to hot, cooked vegetables, potatoes, grilled meat or fish. Plenty of butter can be used on bread or toast. Salad cream or mayonnaise adds calories to salads, potatoes and sandwich fillings.

❖ **Grated cheese.** A bag can be kept in the fridge to put on vegetables, potatoes, soups, scrambled egg, omelette or sauces.

❖ **Evaporated milk/double cream.** Can be used to make savoury dishes such as soups, sauces, casseroles and scrambled egg. Can also be used to make sweet dishes such as custard, added to yoghurt or other instant deserts, or used on breakfast cereals.

❖ **Honey/jam/sugar/syrup.** Add extra to puddings, drinks, fruits, yoghurts, breakfast cereals, bread and toast.

Prescribed supplements

There are no didactic rules for when to introduce prescribed supplements. It is frequently a negotiated issue and seen as a part of caring. Enriching of ordinary food should, however, normally be tried first, as this is often better tolerated.

For patients where prescribed supplements are indicated and wanted, there are three main groups:

⌘ **Calorie supplements,** eg. Maxijul® powder and liquid, Polycal®, Caloreen®, Calsip®. Most come as liquids or powders. They are carbohydrate-based and can be used to enrich other foods.

⌘ **Protein supplements.** These are indicated for hypoproteinaemia.

⌘ **Sip feeds,** eg. Ensure Plus®, Enlive®, Fortisip®, Fresubin®. These contain energy, carbohydrate, fat and protein, with vitamins and trace elements in a nutritionally balanced formulation. They come in cartons and are designed to be sipped, although manufacturers also provide recipe leaflets for sweet and savoury dishes and drinks in which they can be incorporated.

Palatability and patient preference varies. The range of flavours and makes is vast (for example, see *Table 4.5.1*).

Table 4.5.1: Prescribed supplements

Type of supplement	Name	Presentation	Features
Calorie supplements (not nutritionally complete)	Calogen	Bottle 250 ml or 1 litre	High-fat supplement
	Caloreen	Tin 500 g	Glucose polymer
	Calshake	Powder in sachets	Fat/carbohydrate supplement
	Duobar	High-energy bar	Fat/carbohydrate supplement
	Duocal	Supersoluble powder/liquid	Fat/carbohydrate supplement
	Maxijul	Supersoluble powder/liquid	Carbohydrate supplement
	Polycal	Supersoluble powder/liquid	Carbohydrate supplement
	Polycose	Supersoluble powder/liquid	Carbohydrate supplement
	Procal	Sachets	Fat/carbohydrate supplement with protein
	Quickcal	Sachets/tubs	Fat/carbohydrate supplement with protein
	Scandishake		Fat/carbohydrate supplement with protein
	Vitasavoury	Sachets/tubs Powder Sachets/cups	Fat/carbohydrate supplement with protein
Protein supplements (not nutritionally complete)	Casilan 90	Powder	Protein supplement
	Forceval protein	Powder	Protein/carbohydrate supplement
	Maxipro	Powder	Protein supplement
	Promod	Powder (tins)	Protein supplement
	Protifar	Powder	Protein supplement
	Vitapro	Powder	Protein supplement
Sip feeds (some are nutritionally complete)	Clinutren	Liquid in cup or desert	Nutritionally complete
	Enlive	Cartons (fruit)	Not nutritionally complete
	Enrich (Enrich plus)	Cans	Nutritionally complete
	Ensure (Ensure plus)	Cans	Nutritionally complete
	Forticreme	Deserts in pots	Not nutritionally complete
	Fortijuce	Cartons (fruit)	Not nutritionally complete
	Fortimel	Cartons	Not nutritionally complete
	Fortisip	Cartons	Nutritionally complete
	Fresubin	Cartons	Nutritionally complete
	Nutricomp	Cartons/desserts in cups	Nutritionally complete
	Provide xtra		Not nutritionally complete
	Resource shake		Not nutritionally complete
Sip feeds with eicosapentaenoic acid	ProSure	Cartons	See text below

All these supplements are prescribable on a FP10, provided the prescriber endorses the prescription 'ACBS' and the recipient's condition falls within the ACBS indications for that product. 'Borderline substances' are foods that can be prescribed in certain situations. A full list of these products is in the back of the *British National Formulary* (*BNF*) under 'Borderline substances' and in the *Monthly Index of Medical Specialties* (*MIMS*) under 'Tube and sip feeds' and 'Modular supplements'.

It makes sense to prescribe small quantities of an appropriate supplement in a range of flavours and makes until a palatable preparation is found. Some community pharmacists will cooperate with tasting schemes and carry a range of products for that purpose; otherwise, many district nurses set up similar schemes.

Sip feeds with eicosapentaenoic acid

Recent research has identified eicosapentaenoic acid (EPA; a polyunsaturated fatty acid of the omega-3 family derived from fish oils) as a promising agent in modifying the production of pro-inflammatory cytokines. By doing this it is altering the underlying metabolic abnormalities that are believed to produce cancer-associated weight loss. One product (ProSure) incorporates a nutritionally balanced sip feed with EPA. Early results from small trials suggests this combination is effective in moderating cancer-induced weight loss, and this may be a useful agent in the management of these patients.

The manufacturers recommended dose is titration over four days, from half a carton a day to two cartons a day. Clearly, it can only be of benefit with cancer-associated weight loss.

4.6 Enteral and parenteral feeding

Occasionally, oral feeding is not sufficient to support patients' needs. Provided their overall condition warrants it, and they are in agreement, enteral or parenteral feeding may be indicated (*Figure 4.6.1*).

It is beyond the scope of this section to give detailed guidance on regimens. Both enteral and parenteral nutrition can be sustained at home given good cooperation and support from inpatient services, the dietician, the pharmacist, the laboratory services, the GP, the district nurse and the patient and family. Usually this is coordinated from the inpatient service, but the GP and district nurse are key to its success.

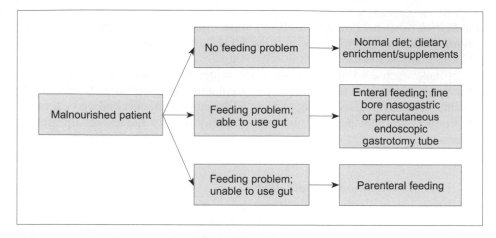

Figure 4.6.1: Indications for enteral or parenteral feeding

4.7 Nutrition as death approaches

One of the commonest features as death approaches is a profound loss of appetite. The patient rarely wants food and may increasingly refuse liquids. This can be a source of much distress to families, but is almost certainly a part of the natural process of dying (see *Chapter 6, p. 114*). Acknowledgement of the family's concern and explanation is vital.

> *I often explain that as the body comes closer to death, it is just too*
> *weak to digest food or take liquid any more. That the energy needs*
> *of the body are so small that the person will not feel hunger, but*
> *if they do to give a sip of soup or a mouthful of something light.*
> *That the body naturally reduces or stops its fluid intake. That this*
> *often increases comfort by reducing secretions: reducing phlegm,*
> *coughing and noisy breathing, reducing the stomach secretions and*
> *any chance of sickness; reducing urine output and the need to toilet.*
> *Most families are happy with this.*

Palliative care specialist

> *All he was having was those drinks, and I'm sure he was drinking*
> *them just to please me. I'm sure he never wanted them, but in my*
> *silly mind he needed them because he needed the strength. What was*
> *the point? He was virtually dying and I was pushing these drinks*
> *down him.*

Woman caring for husband dying of lung cancer at home

Thirst is rare. If it seems to be present it can be quenched with careful mouthcare, such as sips of fluid or a favourite liquid slipped in the mouth on a mouthcare sponge. Occasionally, if thirst is unassailable or patient and family are committed to fluids, subcutaneous fluids can be given slowly through a butterfly needle (see *Chapter 6, Table 6.6.1, p. 123*).

Discontinuing enteral or parenteral nutrition needs careful negotiation with the family, but similar arguments apply in the last few days of life. The percutaneous endoscopic gastrotomy tube or central line can provide another route of access for necessary comfort medication. Removal of the rest of the apparatus is often a great relief, allowing a closer level of physical contact and intimacy.

Key points

❖ Healthcare professionals are concerned with nutrition; patients and families need nourishment. Nutrition is only one aspect of this.
❖ There is considerable evidence that diet and moderate evidence that vitamin supplements play a role in the prevention of cancer. Their role once cancer is established is less clear.
❖ Extreme diets are nutritionally unsound, especially for patients with reduced appetite.
❖ Most patients with reduced appetite can be helped by dietary enrichment and corticosteroids or progestogens.
❖ Where supplements are prescribed, due regard should be paid to the best type of supplement and to patient preference and palatability as compliance is often poor.
❖ Sip feeds with eicosapentaenoic acid are a promising development.
❖ Food and fluid intake diminish naturally as death approaches. This may assist the overall comfort of the dying process.

Further reading

Allwood MC (1999) Stability issues of parenteral nutrition in homecare. *Br J Homecare* **Jan/Feb**: 16–21

Department of Health (1998) *Nutritional Aspects of the Development of Cancer (COMA). Summary of Dietary Recommendations.* Department of Health, London

Goodman S, MacClaren Howard J, Barker W (1994) Nutrition and lifestyle guidelines for people with cancer. *J Nutr Med* **4**: 199–214

Goodman S (2001) The role of nutrition. In: Barraclough J, ed. *Integrated Cancer Care.* Oxford University Press, Oxford

Jatoi A Jr, Loprinz i CL (2001) Current management of cancer-associated anorexia and weight loss. *Oncology* (Huntigt) **15**(4): 497–502

Jatoi A, Daly BD, Kramer G, Mason JB (1998) A cross-sectional study of vitamin intake in post-operative non-small cell lung cancer patients. *J Surg Oncol* **68**(4): 231–6

5

Non-cancer palliative care

5.1 General principles for non-cancer palliative care

Much of the skill and knowledge of specialist palliative care services is derived from working with patients dying of cancer. A good part of the palliative care workload for the primary healthcare team involves non-cancer diagnoses. Primary healthcare teams are in a strong position to coordinate the care of these patients, particularly with a good understanding of both the strengths and limitations of specialist palliative care services for patients with non-cancer diagnoses.

Frequently, patients dying of non-cancer diagnoses receive less coordinated palliative care than patients dying of cancer. We need better systems within primary care for identifying and managing these patients.

Many of the skills and strengths of palliative care that have been derived from cancer patients are readily transferable to all patients with palliative care needs:

- good control of physical symptoms
- multiprofessional approach with good teamwork
- holistic approach, respecting patient's uniqueness
- attention to openness and honesty in communication
- discussion and support for patient and family about end-of-life issues where wanted
- support of family/carers, both practical, educational and emotional
- spiritual support.

The primary care team should:

⌘ Establish a method of identifying this group of patients and the individuals involved in their care (including lay carers).
⌘ Liaise well with specialist services for the disease concerned. This means good communication. Some specialties are developing nurse specialists who are able to develop expertise in palliative aspects of specific diseases, as well as developing joint working with palliative care specialists. Examples are for patients with acquired immunodeficiency syndrome (AIDS), heart failure and motor neurone disease (MND).
⌘ Liaise with specialist palliative care services where necessary. Many

specialist palliative care services can offer support to patients with non-cancer diagnoses, although this is variable, and many differentiate between physical diagnoses and dementias. Most specialist palliative care services can support and advise professionals who are caring for patients dying of non-cancer diagnoses.

⌘ Clarify the roles of different team members.
⌘ Use a palliative care approach. Start with an open question, for example, 'What are your three most troublesome problems?', and consider using a checklist that includes psychological, social and spiritual concerns.
⌘ Identify access to services, such as:
  • specialist community liaison nurses
  • psychological support/counselling
  • community dietician
  • community occupational therapist/physiotherapist
  • district nursing
  • aids/adaptations
  • social worker.
⌘ Address information, education and support needs of patient and family.

5.2 The differences between cancer and non-cancer palliative care

It is important to recognize some fundamental differences:

⌘ Diagnosis of dying is more difficult because the illness trajectory is different (*Figure 5.2.1*). Usually it is longer and more fluctuating. For some non-cancer diagnoses it may also need to contain an awareness of a high chance of sudden death. This creates different patterns of emotional, social and spiritual need. For example, patients with heart failure may suddenly improve, and we are left with the dilemma of how to withdraw care.
⌘ Incidence, duration, type and intensity of symptoms differ.
⌘ There may be less fear/stigma attached to the diagnosis; for example, patients and families may regard heart failure as, 'at least it's not cancer'.
⌘ There may be more fear/stigma, eg. AIDS, Creutzfeld–Jakob's disease (CJD).
⌘ Long-term mental confusion and disability are more common. A dignified death with full control, awareness and choice may prove impossible.
⌘ Patients tend to be older and have additional illnesses.
⌘ Patients may have outlived carers.
⌘ Specialist palliative care teams may not have training/expertise in non-cancer diagnoses.

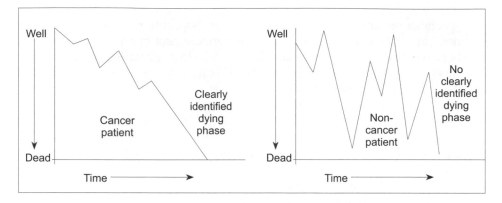

Figure 5.2.1: Typical illness trajectories in patients with and without cancer

5.3 What sort of non-cancer patients may have palliative care needs?

There are clearly many different scenarios, such as:

- end-stage ischaemic heart disease, congestive cardiac failure, peripheral vascular disease
- end-stage chronic obstructive pulmonary disease (COPD), fibrosing alveolitis, cystic fibrosis
- end-stage rheumatoid arthritis
- end-stage MND, multiple sclerosis, cerebral palsy
- end-stage renal failure
- AIDS
- Alzheimer's disease and other dementias
- CJD
- uncertain prognosis/diagnosis
- children with life-limiting disease.

5.4 Terminal care of the elderly

Even with a co-existing cancer diagnosis, there may be specific challenges for older people:

⌘ There is often multisystem disease. This may affect treatment options and produce complex illness trajectories, making prediction unreliable.

⌘ Symptoms may be of longer duration, difficult to palliate and have greater impact on dignity and quality of life, eg. loss of cognitive function, incontinence, loss of mobility may already have been present for some time.

⌘ Dying is more likely to be diagnosed by exclusion.

⌘ This often leads to a short gap between expectation of death and actual death, with little opportunity for preparedness, saying goodbye or anticipatory grieving.

⌘ The absence of a clear 'terminal phase' excludes many older people from palliative care programmes or specialist services.

⌘ Communication may be more difficult because of confusion, dysphasia, poor hearing and vision.

⌘ Reduced social network.

The practice needs to have good links with the elderly care services, social care services and local residential and nursing homes.

5.5 Palliative care and heart failure

Heart failure is often viewed by patients and their families as being a 'better' diagnosis than cancer. Its morbidity and mortality are, however, almost identical (*Table 5.5.1*).

Table 5.5.1: Morbidity and mortality of severe heart failure and cancer

Severe heart failure	Cancer
60% mortality at 1 year	60% mortality at 5 years
70% in hospital during last year of life	90% in hospital during last year of life
54% die in hospital	50% die in hospital
30% die at home	29% die at home

Physical symptoms of heart failure, such as pain, breathlessness, weight loss ('cardiac cachexia'), nausea and vomiting, weakness and incontinence are common, and comparable with the physical symptoms of cancer (*Table 5.5.2*).

The most troublesome symptoms are breathlessness, angina and tiredness. Emotional problems are also common, but not often documented or addressed.

Reduced libido is common (two-thirds of patients in one study).

Despite this, patients with heart failure have little information on or understanding of their diagnosis or prognosis. They often experience poorly coordinated care, less access to benefits and less access to district nursing or specialist community care (*Figure 5.5.1*, opposite).

Table 5.5.2: Prevalence of physical symptoms of cancer and heart disease*

Symptoms	Heart disease	Cancer
Pain	77%	88%
Dyspnoea	60%	54%
Confusion	32%	41%
Constipation	38%	63%
Vomiting	32%	59%
Incontinence	30%	40%

*Adapted from Hall (1996)

Challenges for palliation in heart failure

✤ Counselling may be challenging. Heart failure has a high incidence of sudden death (50%). Patients and families perceive a more benign nature: there is unpredictability, both for sudden death and for the illness trajectory. Patients may appear near-death, yet recover, be sent home apparently well, only to die without warning a short time later. This sort of uncertainty is stressful for everyone concerned. Acknowledging that can help patients, families and the primary care team

✤ Symptom control. Optimal control of the heart failure will maximize symptom control. If breathlessness is severe despite optimal management, small, regular doses of oral morphine will help. Domiciliary oxygen may be helpful. It is worth trying to maintain diuretic therapy even when the patient is too near death to continue oral medications. Furosemide (frusemide) can be given subcutaneously.

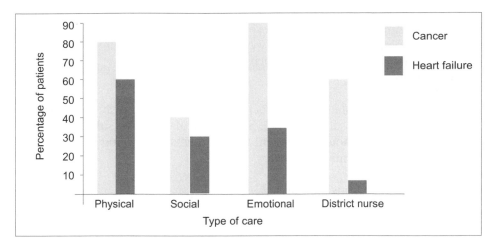

Figure 5.5.1. Patients receiving physical, emotional, social and district nurse care with cancer and heart failure. Adapted from Anderson *et al* (2001)

5.6 Palliative care for end-stage pulmonary disease

End-stage breathlessness from any non-reversible cause responds to the general methods of controlling breathlessness (see *3.4, p. 51*). If standard treatment has failed to give relief and the patient is distressed, small doses of morphine and lorazepam by mouth (or diamorphine and midazolam subcutaneously) can bring comfort. They need to be started cautiously, especially if the patient is thought to have carbon dioxide retention.

Prescribe immediate-release (IR) formulations initially. End-stage respiratory failure is distressing for patients and families. As the oxygen saturation reduces, patients become increasingly anxious, cyanosed and confused, fighting for breath until they lapse into unconsciousness. Progressive central cyanosis despite controlled oxygen therapy is an indicator. Parenteral doses of diamorphine and midazolam, titrated up until the patient is comfortable, will bring ease. If excessive secretions are troublesome, glycopyrollate 0.2 mg every four hours or hyoscine hydrobromide 0.4 mg every four hours combined with positioning and portable suction will help.

5.7 Palliative care for end-stage renal disease

Patients dying of renal failure generally die a gentle, peaceful death, which can be comforting knowledge. Symptoms to anticipate are:

- nausea/vomiting. This usually responds to cyclizine 50 mg subcutaneously three times a day or 150 mg subcutaneously every twenty-four hours in a syringe driver
- hiccoughs
- itch
- multifocal myoclonus or fits. Fits are rare and almost always preceded by widespread muscle twitching. Start midazolam 30 mg subcutaneously over twenty-four hours to prevent fitting; increase in 10 mg over twenty-four-hour increments if necessary.

None of these symptoms are inevitable.

5.8 Palliative care for end-stage neurological disease

Many specialist palliative care services have developed interest and expertise in the end-stage management of motor neurone disease (MND). Some also offer support and help for patients with end-stage multiple sclerosis. Many of these patients, along with patients dying from cerebrovascular disease, Parkinson's disease and cerebral palsy, involve a number of different disciplines and services: neurology, elderly care medicine, young disabled units, general medicine, and so on.

Common problems in end-stage neurological disease

⌘ **Pain:** This may be stiffness and cramp secondary to immobility or muscle spasm. Generally, it responds well to small doses of morphine. Non-steroidal anti-inflammatory drugs may also help. Massage, positioning, heat, cold, physiotherapy and transcutaneous electrical nerve stimulation (TENS) are other options. If there is marked muscle spasm, a muscle relaxant such as diazepam or baclofen may help (although patients sometimes find they have been relying on a degree of muscle spasm to maintain function). Occasionally, botulinus toxin injection can give relief.

⌘ **Nutrition:** There may be difficulties with swallowing, causing nutritional deficit, drooling, coughing and aspiration. Neurological dysphagia generally warrants early discussion of percutaneous endoscopic gastrostomy (PEG) feeding. This can be helpful in improving nutrition, wellbeing and quality of life, but it is not always the right choice if the patient sees it as prolonging an intolerable and deteriorating situation.

This needs careful discussion before the procedure is undertaken; it is a much harder decision for everybody to discontinue PEG feeding than not to start it. Drooling is discussed on *page 79* and the management of cough on *page 57*. Early involvement of the dietitian and dietary enrichment/supplements should be considered (see *Chapter 4, p. 93*).

⌘ **Respiratory problems:** These are a common feature of advanced MND. 'Choking to death' is a common fear for patients and families. Research has shown that almost all patients with MND die peacefully (98%), and over half of these died at home. Patients and families need this information (Neudert *et al*, 2001). General methods for the relief of breathlessness are helpful (see *p. 46*). Morphine and benzodiazepines are beneficial. Home mechanical ventilation is sometimes used. Consider providing a 'breathing-space pack'. These are available through the MND Association, David Niven House, PO Box 246, Northampton NN1 2PR (Telephone 01604 250505). The kit contains a selection of needles and syringes. It needs stocking by the GP with appropriate doses of diamorphine, a benzodiazepine and an antisecretory for rapid administration by patient, family, doctor or nurse in the event of a choking episode (*Table 5.8.1*).

The MND Society pack contains written instructions for the patient, family and carers.

Physiotherapy/speech therapy assessment is important if there is thought to be risk of aspiration. Antibiotics may provide useful palliation in the presence of infection, but this needs to be carefully balanced against the patient's overall quality of life and known wishes.

Table 5.8.1: Doses for contents of the breathing-space pack

Sublingual or	Oramorph concentrated solution 10 mg	Lorazepam 1–2 mg	Hyoscine 0.3 mg tablets
Rectal or	Morphine sulphate or suppository 10 mg	Diazepam (Stesolid) 10mg x3	
Subcutaneous	Diamorphine 5–10 mg 5–10 mg x3	Midazolam 5–10 mg 5–10 mg x3	Hyoscine 0.4 mg injection x3

Dying of end-stage MND and simililar neurological diseases

Severe pain is rare. The most common reported symptoms in patients with MND during the last twenty-four hours were dyspnoea, coughing, anxiety and restlessness. These will usually respond well to diamorphine and midazolam given subcutaneously via a syringe driver. If the patient has not been on opioids before, start with diamorphine 10 mg and midazolam 10 mg every twenty-four hours via a syringe driver. Both of these can be increased in 10 mg increments (or 50% increments at higher doses) until the patient is comfortable. The PEG tube will allow easy administration of additional doses (if in place).

5.9 Palliative care for end-stage dementias

Pain is poorly diagnosed and under-treated in patients with advanced dementia:

- while dementia does not cause pain, patients commonly have co-existing painful conditions
- patients are unable to verbalize pain and other symptoms
- both professional and lay carers are not always sure how to assess pain in the absence of verbal information
- there may be concerns about painkillers causing sedation, increasing confusion, constipation or leading to falls in this group of patients.

Table 5.9.1 lists one approach to assessing pain in patients with advanced dementia.

As a general rule, if you would expect a patient without dementia to experience pain, assume the patient with the same condition with dementia has pain, unless you can prove otherwise. If there is no physical reason for the patient to be experiencing pain and the behaviour changes in *Table 5.9.1* are present, this may be emotional or spiritual pain. Check with the family for recent change or loss. Emotional pain is common in these patients where it becomes so difficult to do even simple tasks. Old photographs, music, massage, companionship and skilled support from specialist dementia services may help. Sometimes an antidepressant may be needed.

There is good evidence that the use of a simple protocol (such as the assessment of discomfort in dementia protocol by Weissman *et al*, 1999) allows more accurate management of both physical and emotional pain in patients with dementia.

Consent to treatment can be a problem with this group of patients. Legally, in the absence of any advanced directive from the patient, treatment may be given if it is judged to be in the patient's best interest. It is important to note that relatives and staff have no legal right to consent on the patient's behalf. Ultimately, the decision lies with the doctor, but the burdens and benefits of any intervention should be carefully considered in consulation with relatives and carers.

There is a high incidence of carer strain and depression with dementia.

Table 5.9.1: Assessing pain in the patient with advanced dementia	
Suspect	Patient has painful co-exiting disease: ❖ arthritis ❖ ischaemic heart disease ❖ cancer ❖ ulcers/pressure sores ❖ infection/inflammation
Most common signs	Patient shows new or increased behavioural signs: ❖ tense posture/body language ❖ sad facial expression ❖ fidgeting ❖ repetitive verbalisations ❖ calling out
Other common signs	❖ increased agitation ❖ repetitive movements ❖ decreased cognition ❖ decreased functional ability ❖ withdrawal ❖ changes in sleep pattern ❖ falling ❖ increase in pulse, blood pressure, and sweating
Treatment	❖ painkillers are introduced in a stepwise way ❖ tolerance is assessed ❖ symptoms usually settle (if not, could this be emotional pain?)

5.10 Palliative care where there is no diagnosis

Sometimes, the primary care team can be caring for someone who is clearly dying, but has not got a definite diagnosis. This produces many challenges:

- working with uncertainty
- balancing vigorous assessment/investigation against overall quality of life
- unpredictable illness trajectory
- trying to anticipate problems and prepare the family
- unclear care pathways/links to specialist services
- death certification/post-mortem.

This sometimes produces many difficulties for families who expect clearer information. Honesty and shared decision-making are paramount.

5.11 Palliative care and AIDS

Much of the underlying philosophy and principles of palliative care are helpful in caring for patients with AIDS secondary to human immunodeficiency virus (HIV) infection. Fundamental to this is the practice of a high standard of scientific medicine alongside a compassionate, whole-person, individualized approach.

Challenges for the primary care team

⌘ Knowing how to access best current practice in anti-retroviral treatments and their common side-effects and interactions. Multiple drug therapy is common and drug interactions are common and potentially serious. Many patients take an active interest in their therapy and become expert, but if in doubt ask your local expert resource.

⌘ Aggressive treatment may be continued until late in the illness, and decisions about the transition from aggressive treatment with best supportive care to a purely palliative management, treatment withdrawal and the management of a potentially prolonged dying phase need to be carefully negotiated.

⌘ Generally, the transition to palliative care will be:
  • when the side-effects of treatment exceed any benefits, or treatment has ceased to be effective
  • if the patient no longer wishes to continue aggressive treatment
  • when vital organs fail.

⌘ Some prophylactic treatment, for example for candidiasis, *pneumocystis carinii* pneumonia, cytomegalovirus or herpes simplex, or anti-tubercular therapy may need to be continued until close to death.

⌘ Patients with AIDS are often younger adults or children. Because of the way it spreads, part or all of a family unit may be affected. The patient may have watched a partner, parent or child die. There may be issues of guilt related to transmission, whether from sexual behaviour, drug abuse, contaminated blood products or childbirth. There may be anger, powerlessness and helplessness. The caregiver may be infected with HIV. There is a need for skilled counselling and social support for patient and family unit, and the primary care team should be aware of how to access local resources.

⌘ HIV and AIDS still carry much stigma, fear, irrational beliefs and practice and isolation. Patients may find it difficult to discuss their illness and death within their family and friendship network, which can increase fear, isolation and unpreparedness for the dying phase. It is still sadly common for fear about the diagnosis or conflict about lifestyle choices or sexual orientation to lead to stress or breakdown of family bonds.

⌘ As with other non-cancer diagnoses, the course is unpredictable. An opportunistic infection may bring the patient close to death, only to recover for an uncertain length of time before another unpleasant and hazardous infection comes.

⌘ The principles of pain and symptom control and the use of the World Health Organization's analgesic ladder are equally applicable in patients with AIDS. Neuropathies may occur both as a symptom of AIDS and as a side-effect of treatment. Tricyclic antidepressants and/or anticonvulsants can be useful adjuvants for management of neuropathic pain, always checking for potential drug interactions. Pain tends to be undertreated compared with cancer. Diarrhoea can be a problem (see *p. 58*). Where there has been lung involvement with tuberculosisor *pneumocystis carinii* pneumonia, standard palliative interventions for breathlessness will help (see *p. 51*). If AIDS-related dementia occurs, the section on dementia above (see *p. 106*), and on confusion (*Chapter 13, p. 176*) may be useful.

⌘ Not all specialist palliative care services have the resource to take patients with infectious illnesses. In large population centres with many patients suffering from AIDS, specialist hospice services are available. These are a useful service nationally as they have developed particular expertise and offer outreach training. Specialist AIDS hospices may present problems for those who wish to maintain confidentiality about their diagnosis. Ability to provide a service for patients with AIDS varies in general hospices, and primary care teams need to check local availability.

⌘ Death certificates are not private documents, and the information on them is publicly available. If confidentiality is an issue, remember that the reason people die from AIDS is because of complications of the disease. It is legitimate to certify death as being caused by pneumonia, encephalopathy or skin cancer, for example, ticking the box that says 'Further information may be available later'. The diagnosis is then recorded for statistical purposes, but is not in the public domain.

⌘ Bodies are potentially infectious for a week after death. Provided the body is sealed in a body bag, with strict instructions that it is not to be opened and may present an infection risk, there is no requirement to inform the undertaker or associated staff of the diagnosis.

Key points

❖ Many of the skills and strengths of palliative care that have been derived from cancer patients are readily transferable to all patients with palliative care needs.

❖ There are some fundamental differences and the specialist palliative care teams may not have training/expertise in non-cancer diagnoses.

❖ Non-cancer illnesses are longer, more fluctuating and the dying phase is often less easy to diagnose.

❖ Non-cancer illnesses may have mortality and morbidity comparable with cancer, but symptom control, communication and support needs are less well coordinated.

❖ The GP is seen as the key worker, and increasingly specialist community liaison nurses are addressing the palliative care aspects of looking after patients with non-cancer diagnoses.

❖ Pain is poorly diagnosed and under-treated in patients with advanced dementia.

❖ As a general rule, if you would expect a patient without dementia to experience pain, assume the patient with the same condition with dementia has pain, unless you can prove otherwise.

References

Anderson H, Ward C, Eardley A, Gomm SA, Connolly M, Coppinger T *et al* (2001) The concerns of patients under palliative care and a heart failure clinic are not being met. *Palliat Med* **15:** 279–86

Hall A (1996) *Managing Terminal Illness*. Royal College of Physicians, London

Weissman D *et al* (1999) Pain management for patients with late-stage dementia. *J Pain Symptom Manage* **18**: 412–19

Further reading

Exerpta Medica MND Advisory Group/Association of British Neurologists (1999) *Guidelines for the Management of Motor Neurone Disease (MND)*. Association of British Neurologists Guidelines. Available online: www.theabn.org/downloads/mnddoc

Hanratty B, Hibbert D, Mair F, Mayu C, Ward C, Capewell S *et al* (2002) Doctors' perceptions of palliative care for heart failure: focus study group. *Br Med J* **325**: 581–5

Jones G, Faull C, Carter Y (1998) Palliative care for people with acquired immune deficiency syndrome (AIDS). In: Faull C, Carter Y, Woof R, eds. *Handbook of Palliative Care*. Blackwell Science Ltd, Oxford: 202–6

Kafetz K (2002) What happens when elderly people die? *J Roy Soc Med* **95**: 536–8

McCarthy M, Hall JA, Ley M (1997) Communication and choice in dying from heart disease. *J Roy Soc Med* **90**: 128–31

Neudert C, Oliver D, Wasner M, Borasio G (2001) The course of the terminal phase in patients with amyotrophic lateral sclerosis. *J Neurol* **248**: 612–16

O'Brien T, Welsh J, Dunn F (1998) Non-malignant conditions. In: Fallon M, O'Neill B, eds. *ABC of Palliative Care*. BMJ Books, London: 54–57

Voltz R, Borasio GD (1997) Palliative therapy in the terminal stage of neurological disease *J Neurol* **244**: S2–10

Wesby PD, Richardson A, Brettle RP (1998) AIDS: aspects in adults. In: Doyle D, Hanks GWC, MacDonald N, eds. *Oxford Textbook of Palliative Medicine*. 2nd edn. Oxford University Press, Oxford: 1121–46

6

Dying — managing the last few days

6.1 A good death — what do we mean?

Dying is an inevitable and universal human experience. All of us wish a good death for ourselves and those we love. What this means in practice and the value given to different aspects of the experience of dying varies widely from person to person. There are wider variations within and between cultural, racial and religious groups and between different generations. A good death could be defined as a death that is congruent with an individual's life; that reflects his or her beliefs and values. As healthcare professionals, we focus on peace, freedom from pain, dignity and family support. These are widely held and laudable goals, provided that we also remember to check that they are shared by the dying person and his or her family. Some patients may value complete clarity of mind above pain control. We have all met individuals who have chosen not to 'go gently into that good night', but to 'fight every inch of the way'.

A death that has gone well is deeply satisfying for the primary healthcare team. It raises morale and can improve team relationships. Conversely, a death that is felt to have gone badly can cause distress and suffering for the doctors and nurses involved, as well as the bereaved family members. Memories of a bad death stay with families for generations and can impact on many future deaths, becoming part of family folklore to be remembered vividly next time by both the dying person and by those caring for him or her (and possibly also by the doctor and nurse if they were involved).

6.2 Diagnosing dying

To be able to optimize care during the dying phase (the last few days of life), we need to be able to recognize and diagnose that the patient is dying. There is surprisingly little research and training about how this is done. Prognostic error, even by highly skilled groups of doctors working in daily contact with cancer or palliative care, is widespread. Doctors tend to be over-optimistic, particularly where they know their patients well. Sometimes families or untrained nursing staff appreciate the reality of the situation first. The transition from the palliative phase to the dying phase of the journey may also be more readily recognized by an uninvolved, though experienced clinician.

Table 6.2.1 lists some clinical situations that tend to mean life expectancy is short (one to two weeks).

Table 6.2.1: Situations suggesting the last week or two of life[*]
Hypercalcaemia unresponsive to treatment
Bone marrow failure without blood/platelet transfusions
Disseminated intravascular coagulation
Liver metastases with severe jaundice
Progressive renal failure
Chest infection in a frail, bedbound patient
Some forms of cancer carry a short prognosis, such as disseminated adenocarcinoma from an unknown primary
*Adapted from guidelines on estimating prognosis, with kind permission from Dr Cornelius Woelk and Dr Mike Harlos Manitoba, Canada

Performance status

Performance status (how much the patient can do) is the most consistent predictor of prognosis. Unless there is another correctable cause, progressive weakness and loss of function correlates with short survival time. Initially the patient may struggle with the stairs, then with walking on the level. Transferring from bed to chair to commode becomes an effort needing aids, one person, and then two or more helpers. Eventually the patient becomes bedbound, and may lose the strength to sit even in bed. Gentle enquiry into these markers of function can establish the rate of loss of function. If the patient is deteriorating rapidly (day by day), the prognosis is likely to be days, particularly if they are already bedbound. If the deterioration is slower (week by week), the patient may have several weeks left. Although one can broadly estimate survival from the illness trajectory like this, sometimes a rapid deterioration can supervene (*Table 6.2.2*).

Table 6.2.2: Physical changes suggesting the last few days of life	
Mobility	Extremely weak (history of progression)
	Bedbound
	Need help with all care
Appearance	May be gaunt/cachexic
Behaviour	Drowsy/reduced cognition
	Disorientated place/time
	Difficulty concentrating
	Difficulty cooperating with carers
Oral intake	Very much reduced intake of:
	❖ food
	❖ fluids
Medication	May be unable to take oral medication

Steps to consider when diagnosing dying

⌘ The patient has a diagnosis that is known to lead to death, for which no further active treatment is possible.

⌘ The patient is deteriorating and the multiprofessional team agree the patient is dying.

⌘ There is no correctable cause for the deterioration in the patient's condition.

⌘ The clinical picture corresponds with *Table 6.2.2*, above.

Most of this work has been done on patients with cancer, which has a relatively predictable functional decline. It is not clear how transferable it is to illnesses such as stroke or heart disease, which can follow a much more fluctuating course.

6.3 Goals of care during the dying phase

Sometimes I get wrecked with panic that there are things he needs that I am not aware of because I'm not a nurse. I asked the nurse about him going into hospital for a couple of days. He was very tactful, he said, 'How would you feel if he was going into hospital and time was short?' There was a big pause because I wasn't sure what he was getting at, and then I realised; I said, 'Do you mean you think time is short?' and he said, 'Yes, I think you may only have him for a few more days'. So that was it then, whether they wanted him in hospital or not they weren't going to get him. He was staying where he was within the bosom of his family.

Woman caring for husband dying of lung cancer at home.

Even for a patient who has been treated palliatively for some time, once it is recognized that the patient is dying there is a shift to more 'global' goals of care.

Usually, goals of care will emphasize physical comfort, peace, dignity, spiritual care and care of the family (*Table 6.3.1*).

Example

A patient may have a pain problem that might possibly respond to a complex palliative care intervention such as a nerve block, but this can only be offered in an inpatient setting. Overall, both patient and family wish her to die at home, and she is clearly deteriorating quickly day by day. The wish to die at home matters more than complete pain relief. You might discuss this with her and her family, explaining that you will do everything possible to honour her wishes, but this may mean the pain relief being less good than you hoped, and even then to get relief you may need to increase the opioid to a dose where she is more sleepy than she had wanted. She and her family can then make a choice, which only they can truly make, as care goals at the time of dying are complex and unique.

Table 6.3.1: Key care goals during the last few days of life

Recognizing that the patient is dying and communicating this with the family and professional team

Optimizing physical comfort in accordance with the wishes of patient and family

Minimizing unnecessary and invasive medical or nursing interventions in the last days of life (this includes blood tests, invasive bowel care and turning regimens)

Optimizing day-by-day communication between the professional team members, the out-of-hours services and the lay carers

Family support: practical and emotional

Emotional, spiritual and, where appropriate, religious support

6.4 Decisions around place of death

Ideally, decisions around place of death will already have been discussed. Choices are between death at home and death in an inpatient setting. Inpatient settings include hospices, community hospitals, nursing homes, hospital-based palliative care units and acute hospital wards. Access to appropriate inpatient beds can sometimes be difficult, and depends on local availability, current bed state and patient/family preference.

Hospices

Hospices offer high standards of symptom control, nursing input, emotional and spiritual support and often follow up into bereavement. Not all hospices admit patients twenty-four hours a day, and dying patients, particularly if they are not already known to the hospice team, may not be given as high a priority as patients with symptom control problems. There may also be variations in the ability of hospices to admit patients dying from non-cancer diagnoses or from acquired immunodeficiency syndrome (AIDS). Usually admission needs to be pre-arranged and hospice or specialist staff may wish to assess the patient first. If this is the preferred place of death, advance planning with the hospice team is strongly advised. This also enables the patient and family to be introduced to the idea of hospice care, the care environment and the hospice staff before the dying process starts.

Community hospitals

Where community hospitals are available, they can offer advantages:

- low technology environment
- access to trained nursing staff/medication/equipment
- quieter than acute hospitals
- closer and more convenient for family visiting and support
- continuity of care for the GP practice
- twenty-four-hour access to admissions may be available.

Staffing levels are lower than in hospices, and staff may be less skilled in communication and symptom control. There is evidence that carer satisfaction with community hospital care is greater than for acute hospitals, and if an inpatient hospice bed is not accessible, a community hospital may provide a useful alternative.

Nursing homes

Nursing homes offer some of the advantages of community hospitals. Some offer particular expertise in terminal care. Access to places is often limited, standards vary widely and both patients and families may have emotional resistance to the idea of 'being put in a home'. As well as waiting lists, there are also significant financial implications. Some areas are working hard to improve standards of care for dying patients in nursing homes, targeting specific educational initiatives at them; a version of the Liverpool integrated care pathway for dying patients suitable for nursing home use is available.

Acute hospitals

Acute hospitals remain the setting where most patients in the UK die. Admission in the last few days of life is increasingly to an emergency medical admission unit, which is not an ideal care environment for a dying patient and family. It may be possible to improve the experience by:

- trying to negotiate direct admission to a quieter part of the hospital
- trying to speak directly to a sympathetic consultant or senior member of the medical team
- sending as much detailed information about diagnosis as possible with the patient
- explaining in the admission letter that the patient is dying
- giving clear details of medication administered and contents of syringe driver
- giving clear details of any expressed wishes of patient and family, such as not to be resuscitated and advance directives.

Home

In the UK only one-quarter of cancer deaths and one-fifth of non-cancer deaths occur at home. This means there is a real risk of the primary healthcare team losing skills in this area. If this happened, it would be a huge loss as 60–90% of the population would choose to die at home if possible. Dying at home offers a degree of intimacy with loved ones, a sense of being surrounded by the dear and familiar, and a degree of autonomy and self-control for both patient and family that cannot be reproduced in any other care environment.

Why do so many people who wish to die at home die in other care settings?

Dying at home is associated with:

- having a carer
- stating a preference for dying at home
- being aware of the prognosis and having realistic coping strategies
- having adequate practical community support
- having special equipment.

The commonest reasons for an unwanted admission are related to:

- physical deterioration, especially loss of mobility and/or confusion
- carer fatigue and stress.

Surprisingly, pain and symptom control are not a major cause of a terminal admission. The big gap appears to be access to enough practical home help. This is likely to become more of a problem as the population ages, family size decreases and single-person households increase.

The physical and emotional demands of caring twenty-four-hours-a-day for a loved one who is dying cannot be overestimated. Despite this, most carers report it a satisfying or rewarding experience. Carer satisfaction is generally much higher than after death in an acute hospital. In a number of areas, primary care nurses and doctors are involved with stimulating the development of additional practical homecare services for this group of patients.

If patient and family wish the death to be at home, the practicality of this needs to be addressed

If a home birth was being prepared for, there would be detailed, proactive planning. Generally this would include attention to:

- the care environment
- the lay carers
- the professional carers
- the safety net in case of problems
- anticipating and planning for common problems
- rapid, easy access to medication (including out of hours)
- rapid, easy access to necessary equipment (including out of hours)
- rapid, easy access to medical and nursing staff (including out of hours)
- information and support for patient and carers.

The same careful, detailed approach and proactive planning can transform a death at home into a positive and immensely rewarding service for the primary care team to offer.

⌘ **The care environment:** Nursing a bedbound patient generally presents fewer challenges than nursing a weak patient who is still struggling to transfer to the toilet, commode or chair. The choice of room will generally be what works best for family and nursing staff (*Table 6.4.1*). Check there is access to:
  - a telephone (or mobile phone)
  - facilities for personal care
  - an intercom, baby monitor or handbell for attracting attention.

Table 6.4.1: Choice of room for care of the dying patient

	Advantages	Disadvantages
Upstairs	Familiar bed/bedroom	May be distressing for partner after death
	Usually easy to sleep with partner (double bed)	Difficult if hospital bed/airwave mattress required; may sleep better alone
	Bathroom usually upstairs	Carer needs to come up and downstairs frequently
	Quiet	
Downstairs	Less isolated	Less privacy
	Often more space for bed/mattress/equipment	Unfamiliar sleeping environment
	Easier to monitor by day for partner	Needs a trustworthy call system at night if carer sleeping upstairs
	More a part of everyday activity	May be noisy; difficult to separate from visitors

---

⌘ **The carers:** Nursing a loved one through the last days of his or her life can be a great gift or a terrible burden. Assess the carer(s). Do they:

  - feel able to do it ?
  - have adequate physical strength?
  - have adequate emotional resource?
  - have access to practical help? This may be a rota of carers from within the family network or may need supplementing by district

nurses, home carers, Marie Curie nurses, hospice-at-home nurses or other support schemes
- know what help is available and how to access it? It is best if this is checked out of the patient's hearing, so the carer can speak honestly if he/she has doubts or concerns.

⌘ **The professional support:** Caring for a patient dying at home is demanding of medical and nursing time, and the multiprofessional team need to discuss the situation, the care environment and the carer support available and how much input they can give. The most common reason for admission at this stage is not a lack of expert knowledge, but a lack of hands-on nursing help.

Potential sources of professional help:

- district nursing services
- Marie Curie nursing services can provide one-to-one shifts of nursing care in the home. May be limited to some nights each week, depending on local resource. May also be limited to cancer patients only
- Macmillan carer schemes (can put 'sitters' into the home for varying periods to allow main carer respite)
- Hospice-at-Home schemes (vary considerably from advice/support visits from trained palliative care nurses to schemes able to provide full shifts of palliative nursing care in the home. Skill range varies. Freestanding services or linked to inpatient hospices. Some offer medical advice/ support)
- specialist palliative care community nurse (Macmillan nurse). Does not usually provide hands-on nursing input, but an important resource for the primary care team, patient and family in providing expert advice and emotional support. Usually knowledgeable about local resources and networks.

I cared for him at home, I knew it was what he would want. He was virtually hospital-phobic; he did not like the place at all. He almost never went to a doctor so there was no way I was going to put him into the care of a hospital and know that he wasn't comfortable with it. Besides, it just seemed the normal, natural thing to do, to nurse him at home with his family round him. We had two downstairs rooms, fortunately, so we just moved his bed downstairs and it was OK. I think it was the last ten days that he wasn't able to walk any more. It wasn't easy, but the bathroom is downstairs so he only had to cross the hall to use the loo. They did say they would send nurses in the night if I wanted them and gave the number of the out-of-hours doctor. Between them, that's how we managed until the end.

Woman caring for husband dying of lung cancer at home.

6.5 Safety nets

The physical and emotional strain can quickly become overwhelming, and it is vital that good safety nets are built into the care package. These may range from an agreement that the family will accept more nursing support, to a backup bed being available nearby. In practice, this is rarely needed. However, the family need to know that if the patient needs admitting when they are near death, there is a chance they may die in the ambulance. Conversely, they also need to know that an admission in the last week or two of life may mean the patient becoming too ill to transfer home to die, even if this is their preference.

6.6 Anticipating and planning for common problems at home

Many problems in the last days of life can be predicted and prepared for (see *Table 6.6.1*). Our knowledge of the likely problems enables us to anticipate and plan for appropriate medical and nursing interventions. Each day or each visit, aim as you leave to anticipate what might happen over the next day or two. This includes the following considerations.

Medication

Ensure easy access to medication that is likely to be needed. Consider:

⌘ Keeping a 'palliative care bag' in the practice, containing a syringe driver, needles, tubing and drugs most often used during the dying phase. A prescribing protocol could be put with it as an *aide memoir*. In the event of a sudden deterioration, the bag is taken to the patient's home.
⌘ Leaving a box of injectable medication in the home a week or two before it is needed.
⌘ Leaving the syringe driver in the home before it is needed.
⌘ Working with community pharmacists to carry core drugs most often used during the dying phase. These can then be accessed quickly using the 'urgent' prescription scheme (a standard NHS prescription form marked **urgent** by the doctor).
⌘ Ensuring the '*core four*' are rapidly available — diamorphine, cyclizine, hyoscine hydrobromide and midazolam (*Table 6.6.2*).

Other useful drugs are haloperidol and levomepromazine (see 'A brief guide to drugs for the syringe driver', *p. 144*).

Equipment

Ensure easy access to equipment that is likely to be needed. This includes:

- a hospital style bed/electronic bed
- pressure-relieving mattresses
- commode
- catheterization pack
- intercom
- nebuliser
- syringe driver.

Access and equipment sources vary. Find out where yours are before you need them. Voluntary hospices, hospice-at-home services and community palliative care services may be interested in working with you to set up rapid access loan systems in your area.

Nursing care

Discontinue non-vital nursing interventions. These usually include:

- enemas/suppositories
- checking of temperature, blood pressure or other vital signs
- four-hourly turning regimens.

Areas of care to focus on are:

- nursing on a high-dependency mattress and turning for comfort only
- care of the eyes (regular instillation of artificial tears if open)
- care of the mouth (see *pp. 76–8*)
- personal care to maintain dignity/comfort only
- continence needs (pads, catheter)
- monitoring symptom control/medication
- carer support.

Table 6.6.1: Anticipating and preparing for problems at home

Anticipated problem	Consider and plan
Loss of mobility Unable to transfer safely	• Generally safer and more manageable to nurse in bed • Consider loan of hospital bed/monkey pole/cot sides/commode/urine bottles • Assess for pressure area care and implement appropriate strategy • Indwelling urinary catheter/sheath for men if more acceptable if incontinent/unable to transfer to commode • Bowel care
Loss of ability to eat	• Prepare family and patient for this happening • Explain it is a natural process • Forcing food may create discomfort if too weak to swallow/digest
Loss of ability to drink	• Prepare family and patient for this happening • Explain it is a natural process and may aid comfort by reducing secretions/gastric secretions and chance of vomiting/urine output • Encourage sips/mouth care • If still distressed by thirst, consider subcutaneous fluids (N saline 1 litre over 12 hours via a butterfly into anterior abdominal wall or thigh)*
Loss of ability to swallow	• Convert essential medications to subcutaneous route (if no syringe driver available, see *Table 6.6.2* for alternative strategies)
Delirium and agitation	• Common at the end of life • Distressing and frightening for all involved (see *pp. 87–8*) • Haloperidol 5–30 mg subcutaneously every 24 hours and/or midazolam 5–60 mg every 24 hours (if agitation only)
Pain	• Diamorphine subcutaneously as required in proportion to overall opioid requirement (can be administered sublingually if injection not appropriate) • Leave pre-drawn-up syringes. Leave a subcutaneous indwelling butterfly needle
Vomiting	• Cyclizine 50 mg subcutaneously three times a day or • Buccastem 3 mg sublingual or • Transdermal hyoscine
Dyspnoea	• Common and frightening • Diamorphine, preferably subcutaneously (or sublingually), titrated-up as for pain • Midazolam 2–10 mg subcutaneously or sublingually as required, or 5–30 mg subcutaneously every 24 hours for breathlessness/fear or • Diazepam
Excess respiratory secretions	• Positioning/portable suction (if available) • Hyoscine 0.4 mg sublingually or subcutaneously every 4 hours as required or • Hyoscine 1.6–2.4 mg every 24 hours subcutaneously or • Hyoscine transdermal patch
Changing breathing pattern	• Explanation to family 'He may appear to stop breathing for a time, then draw another breath'

Adapted from *Guidelines on Managing Predictable Problems in Home Death*, with kind permission from Dr Mike Harlos, Manitoba, Canada.
*N saline, 4% dextrose/0.18% saline or 5% dextrose are all suitable. No more than 2 litres/24 hours should be infused into any one site. Fluid should not be pumped in.

Table 6.6.2: The 'core four' drugs for the last days of life

Core four indications in the last days of life	Core four drugs for the last days of life	Alternatives*
Pain or emergency	Rx diamorphine injection: dose 5–10 mg or one-sixth of current 24-hour diamorphine requirement	*Sublingual diamorphine 10 mg or morphine-concentrated liquid 20 mg/5 ml sublingually
Nausea/vomiting	Rx cyclizine injection 50 mg	Buccal prochlorperazine 3 mg/ rectal prochlorperazine 5 mg
Excess secretions	Rx hyoscine hydrobromide injection 0.4 mg	Hyoscine transdermal patch 1 mg every 72 hours (may need 2–3)
Agitation/restlessness	Rx midazolam injection 10 mg	*Sublingual lorazepam 1mg/ rectal diazepam 10 mg

*Sublingual administration is not always easy for patients if the mouth is dry, coordination is poor and cognitive function is reduced. Rectal administration can be a challenge for carers both physically (turning and positioning the patient) and emotionally.

6.7 Carer support and basic information needs

Basic information for lay carers on how to care for very ill patients and how to access help if needed is not given often enough (see *Table 6.7.1*).

Table 6.7.1. Information checklist for carers

Do the family understand the patient is dying?

Do they have any questions about this?

Do they understand the role and purpose of any medication?

Do the family have a written medication regimen they can check with?

Do the family know what medication they can administer themselves and when to call for help?

Do they understand the reduced need for food and fluid?

Do the family know how to turn the patient, if he or she needs moving between nursing visits?

Do the family know how to cope with basic care — washing, toilet needs, care of the mouth and eyes? How much of this do they wish to do themselves? How much nursing help do they need?

Is the care package appropriate and clear?

Do the family have written contact details for nursing and medical services, including any variations out of hours?

Do the family know who/when to contact if problems arise, or after the death?

Do the family have written information available on what to do after a death, local death registration facilities and their opening hours, and local bereavement support services?

6.8 Which drugs to continue in the last few days of life?

The general principles of which drugs to continue in the last few days of life include the following.

Continue essential medication

This means:

- regular, adequate analgesia
- anticonvulsants
- benzodiazepines/phenothiazines.

If your patient becomes unable to swallow:

- morphine by mouth can be replaced by subcutaneous diamorphine. Divide the oral morphine dose (mg) by three to get the equivalent subcutaneous diamorphine dose (mg)
- anticonvulsants can be replaced by diazepam 10–20 mg rectally three times a day or midazolam 30 mg subcutaneously over twenty-four hours
- benzodiazepines/phenothiazines can be given rectally or parenterally.

Discontinue non-essential medication

This may mean:

- steroids
- non-steroidal anti-inflammatory drugs (increase morphine or use suppositories)
- antibiotics
- insulin/oral hypoglycaemics
- antidepressants
- bronchodilators
- anti-hypertensive/anti-arrhythmics
- diuretics (unless severe heart failure)
- laxatives
- iron and vitamin supplements.

Anticipate problems

⌘ Have something available for emergency administration, such as a haemorrhage or fit. Midazolam 10 mg is suitable.
⌘ Use hyoscine hydrobromide **early** to prevent a 'death rattle'; hyoscine hydrobromide 0.4 mg subcutaneously every four hours is suitable.

If your patient is restless check:

• bedclothes are loose
• position is comfortable
• bladder is empty
• rectum is empty
• pain control is adequate
• does he/she have unfinished things to say/do?
• midazolam 30–60 mg subcutaneously every twenty-four hours gives good sedation.

6.9 Communication within the primary care team

Different professionals from different teams may be involved in care during the last few days of life. There may be different partners from the practice, different shifts of nurses, 'out-of-hours' teams for both medical and nursing staff, 'Hospice-at-Home' or Marie Curie nurses, Macmillan or other specialist community palliative care nurses, home carers, community occupational therapy input and so on. This can give excellent seamless care and support, or become a communication quagmire, with conflicting messages and unnecessary duplication (or omission) of key tasks. To avoid this:

⌘ Keep a basic communication sheet in the home. At the very least, this needs to list medications and nursing care plan; ideally it should also carry information about the diagnosis, the information given to patient and family and what is known of the patient's wishes.
⌘ Explore with your out-of-hours service, access to out-of-hours palliative care drugs, syringe drivers and communication forms. This helps them, you and your patients.
⌘ Consider the use of an evidence-based care pathway, such as the Liverpool integrated care pathway for the dying patient. This combines a structured assessment tool, holistic evidence-based care during dying and after death for patient and family with a multidisciplinary record. Using

this tool provides outcomes of care in general settings that are as good as those achieved in a specialist hospice setting.

6.10 Spiritual and religious needs

Patients may have specific religious needs as death approaches. Generally, even if you think you are familiar with aspects of a particular religious practice, it is much better to ask than to assume. A general overview of the diversity of practice is given in *Chapter 21 (pp. 243–9)*.

Spiritual need is universal. This is a time for medical and nursing care to be delivered with the utmost kindness, compassion and respect for the individual who is dying, and the soon-to-be bereaved family.

Remember

Doctors worry about drugs and prescribing. For patients and their families this is the first and only time they will travel through this experience. They worry about practicalities of daily life: drug administration, fluids, food, washing, incontinence, vomiting, mouthcare, practical nursing support and whether they are doing 'the right thing'.

It cannot be stressed enough that family members may be frightened, exhausted, grief-filled and unfamiliar with the natural process of dying. Explain everything several times and ensure clarity about who to call and when; how to contact out-of hours medical and nursing services and the additional sources of help and advice in your area (Macmillan nurses, local hospice advice lines, hospice-at-home services, Marie Curie services). Gently clarify the procedure for after the death; who to phone and when, is often enough at this stage. Written information can be an important back-up. Carers will not always recall the detail of what they have been told.

Key points

❖ Different patients will have different ideas of what constitutes a good death.

❖ The diagnosis of dying is difficult, but there are clear clinical situations that indicate the last two weeks or last few days of life.

❖ Performance status (how much the patient can do) is the most consistent predictor of prognosis.

❖ Goals of care in the dying phase become more general and emphasise physical comfort, peace, dignity, spiritual care and care of the family.

❖ Most people would prefer to die at home, but most die in hospital.

❖ Hospital admission is more often linked to care breakdown than the need for specialist help in symptom control.

❖ Preparation, anticipation and multidisciplinary working are the keys to good care at home.

❖ Ensure rapid access to the 'core four' drugs: diamorphine, cyclizine, hyoscine, hydrobromide and midazolam.

❖ Ensure good information sharing between carers, family and professionals.

Further reading

Brockbank J (2002) What relevance do community hospital beds have for palliative care patients? *Eur J Palliat Care* **9**: 164–6

Chritakis NA, Lamont EB (2000) Extent and determinants of error in doctors' prognoses in terminally ill patients: prospective cohort study. *Br Med J* **320**: 469–73

Ellershaw J, Foster A, Murphy D, Shea T, Overill S *et al* (1997) Development of a multiprofessional care pathway for the dying patient. *Eur J Palliat Care* **4**: 203–8

Ellershaw J, Ward C (2002) Care of the dying patient: the last hours or days of life. *Br Med J* **326**: 30–4

Higginson IJ, Astin P, Dolan S (1998) Where do cancer patients die? *Palliat Med* **12**: 353–63

Hinton J (1996) Services given and help perceived during home care for terminal cancer. *Palliat Med* **10**:125–34

Karlsen S, Addington Hall J (1998) How do cancer patients who die at home differ from those who die elsewhere? *Palliat Med* **12**: 279–86

Thomas K (2000) Out-of-hours palliative care — bridging the gap. *Eur J Palliat Care* **7**: 22–5

Checklist for the last few days of life at home		
Checklist	Yes	No
Has the patient's condition been discussed with the carers?		
Has the patient's medication been reviewed and non-essential medication discontinued?		
Has appropriate medication been prescribed for pain, agitation, nausea/vomiting and excess secretions? (The core four)		
Have all inappropriate interventions been stopped?		
Is the patient nursed on a high-dependency mattress and turned for comfort only?		
Is there a syringe driver available should it be required?		
Are out of hours medical and nursing services aware of the situation?		
Is the carer clear about what medication to give the patient and when?		
Is the carer clear about their role with other nursing care?		
Does the carer know who to contact if the patient's symptoms are not controlled?		

Adapted from *Checklist for the Few Last Days of Life* with permission from Maureen Brown, Derwentside Primary Care Trust, Co Durham

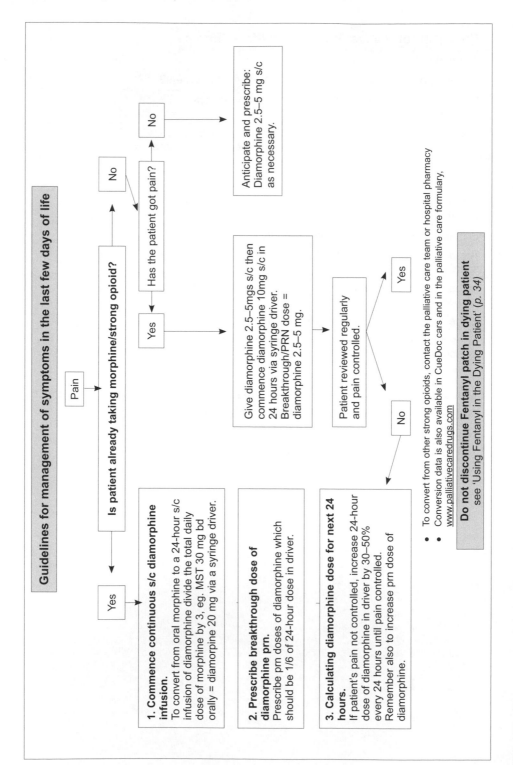

Guidelines for management of symptoms in the last few days of life

Pain

Is patient already taking morphine/strong opioid?

Yes → (to box 1)

No →

Has the patient got pain?

No → Anticipate and prescribe: Diamorphine 2.5–5 mg s/c as necessary.

Yes → Give diamorphine 2.5–5mgs s/c then commence diamorphine 10mg s/c in 24 hours via syringe driver. Breakthrough/PRN dose = diamorphine 2.5–5 mg.

→ Patient reviewed regularly and pain controlled.

Yes

No →

1. Commence continuous s/c diamorphine infusion.
To convert from oral morphine to a 24-hour s/c infusion of diamorphine divide the total daily dose of morphine by 3, eg. MST 30 mg bd orally = diamorpine 20 mg via a syringe driver.

2. Prescribe breakthrough dose of diamorphine prn.
Prescribe prn doses of diamorphine which should be 1/6 of 24-hour dose in driver.

3. Calculating diamorphine dose for next 24 hours.
If patient's pain not controlled, increase 24-hour dose of diamorphine in driver by 30–50% every 24 hours until pain controlled. Remember also to increase prn dose of diamorphine.

- To convert from other strong opioids, contact the palliative care team or hospital pharmacy
- Conversion data is also available in CueDoc cars and in the palliative care formulary, www.palliativecaredrugs.com

Do not discontinue Fentanyl patch in dying patient
see 'Using Fentanyl in the Dying Patient' *(p. 34)*

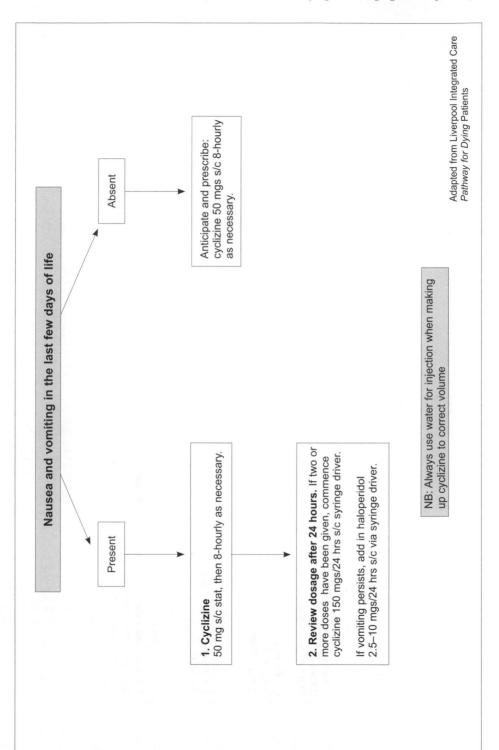

Nausea and vomiting in the last few days of life

Present

Absent

1. Cyclizine
50 mg s/c stat, then 8-hourly as necessary.

2. Review dosage after 24 hours. If two or more doses have been given, commence cyclizine 150 mgs/24 hrs s/c syringe driver.

If vomiting persists, add in haloperidol 2.5–10 mgs/24 hrs s/c via syringe driver.

Anticipate and prescribe: cyclizine 50 mgs s/c 8-hourly as necessary.

NB: Always use water for injection when making up cyclizine to correct volume

Adapted from Liverpool Integrated Care *Pathway for Dying* Patients

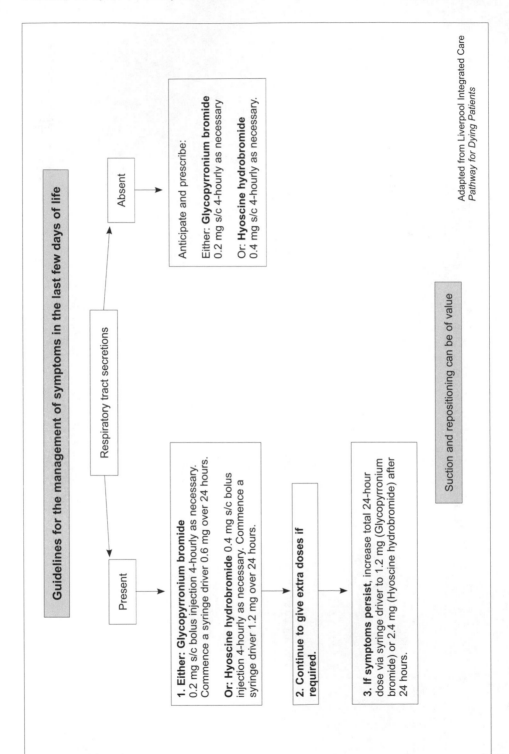

Guidelines for the management of symptoms in the last few days of life

Respiratory tract secretions

Present

Absent

1. **Either: Glycopyrronium bromide**
0.2 mg s/c bolus injection 4-hourly as necessary.
Commence a syringe driver 0.6 mg over 24 hours.

Or: Hyoscine hydrobromide 0.4 mg s/c bolus
injection 4-hourly as necessary. Commence a
syringe driver 1.2 mg over 24 hours.

2. **Continue to give extra doses if
required.**

3. **If symptoms persist,** increase total 24-hour
dose via syringe driver to 1.2 mg (Glycopyrronium
bromide) or 2.4 mg (Hyoscine hydrobromide) after
24 hours.

Anticipate and prescribe:

Either: **Glycopyrronium bromide**
0.2 mg s/c 4-hourly as necessary

Or: **Hyoscine hydrobromide**
0.4 mg s/c 4-hourly as necessary.

Suction and repositioning can be of value

Adapted from Liverpool Integrated Care
Pathway for Dying Patients

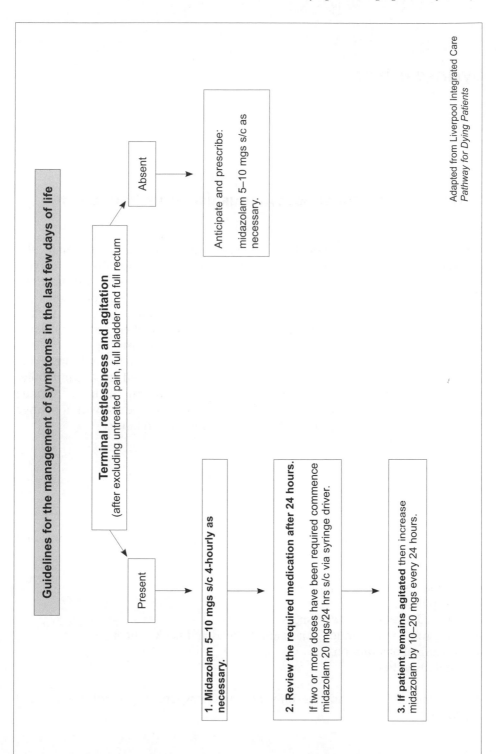

Guidelines for the management of symptoms in the last few days of life

Terminal restlessness and agitation
(after excluding untreated pain, full bladder and full rectum

Present

Absent

Anticipate and prescribe:

midazolam 5–10 mgs s/c as necessary.

1. Midazolam 5–10 mgs s/c 4-hourly as necessary.

2. Review the required medication after 24 hours.

If two or more doses have been required commence midazolam 20 mgs/24 hrs s/c via syringe driver.

3. If patient remains agitated then increase midazolam by 10–20 mgs every 24 hours.

Adapted from Liverpool Integrated Care
Pathway for Dying Patients

7

Syringe drivers

Syringe drivers for subcutaneous use in palliative care

The syringe driver is a portable, battery-operated device for mechanically delivering drugs at a predetermined rate by continuous infusion. Syringe drivers are commonly used for the administration of subcutaneous infusion of drugs. This enables control of symptoms by delivering a constant dose of medication over a twenty-four-hour period via the subcutaneous route. Drugs frequently administered this way include opioid analgesics, anti-emetics, sedatives, some non-steroidal anti-inflammatory drugs and anti-secretory drugs.

Syringe drivers have helped transform the delivery of palliative care in the home setting. However, they are no good in isolation, and need community nursing services trained in their use. Becoming familiar with the use of syringe drivers is a vital palliative care skill. The regular review needed with a syringe driver often brings a structure to the care that improves quality.

Using a syringe driver

The syringe driver should be used when the patient is unable to take oral medication. This may be because of:

- intractable nausea and/or vomiting
- dysphagia
- altered level of consciousness
- oral route not tolerated, for example head and neck cancer
- intestinal obstruction
- malabsorption.

The syringe driver is not the only alternative where oral medication is not appropriate:

- rectal, sublingual or transdermal routes may sometimes be more appropriate, particularly for the ambulatory patient
- if the patient is near death (a couple of hours), one or two four-hourly subcutaneous injections may suffice and be less obtrusive than introducing new technology in the last few hours of life
- if there is likely to be any delay in accessing and setting up the syringe driver, a single subcutaneous injection should be given. This needs to be repeated four-hourly until the syringe driver is running
- if the patient is comfortable and has not needed medication for comfort, there is no need to set up a syringe driver 'just in case' (although it remains important to ensure that there is rapid access to the 'core four' drugs for care during dying should they be needed — diamorphine, cyclizine, hyoscine hydrobromide and midazolam).

A syringe driver is only an alternative method of administering medication. It does not produce more effective analgesia than the oral route unless the patient cannot use oral medication or has serious compliance problems. It does not need to be routinely used as a 'medical last rite' if there is no specific indication for medication.

Setting up a syringe driver

Using guidelines and protocols

Many areas have local guidelines and protocols for syringe driver use. These have arisen because of concerns over consistency, non-standardization of equipment, training, maintenance, prescribing and so on. Where local guidelines or protocols are available, the primary care team should access and follow them.

Specialist palliative care services can usually advise on local guidelines. They can also provide information about training.

Types of syringe driver

Different types of syringe driver are used in different areas. This often causes confusion and sometimes causes serious hazard when staff move from one area to another.

It is vitally important to check the model of syringe driver you are using, to ensure you are familiar with it and to follow the manufacturer's guidelines for that model carefully. If you are not sure, give single doses of any necessary medication and check. The information below refers to the Graseby MS16A and the Graseby MS26 syringe drivers, which are the most common models used in the UK.

The Grasby MS16A (blue syringe driver) is set at mms per hour

The Graseby MS26 (green syringe driver) is set at mms per day

These syringe drivers are calibrated to administer the syringe contents over twenty-four hours +/- 5%. In practice, this means that the syringe driver will empty the syringe in +/- 72 minutes of the expected completion time.

Who sets the syringe driver up?

Only registered nurses and medical practitioners who have been instructed and who are competent should set up a syringe driver. In primary care, syringe drivers are usually set up by district nurses. This can leave a challenge out of hours if there is no access to twenty-four-hour district nursing or community palliative care nursing services.

If a competent healthcare professional is not available, an indwelling subcutaneous butterfly needle will enable the administration of regular doses of prescribed medication until the syringe driver can be set up.

Choosing the skin site

The best sites to use for continuous subcutaneous infusions are:

- the upper chest wall below the clavicle
- the upper arm and thigh
- the abdomen
- occasionally the back
- **avoid**, if possible, the upper arms and outer aspect of the thighs in bed-bound patients requiring turning.

Skin sites not to be used:

- lymphoedematous limbs: the subcutaneous tissues are 'waterlogged' with lymph fluid, which would affect absorption. There is also a risk of leakage and infection
- any site over a bony prominence or near a joint
- the upper abdomen in a patient with an enlarged liver (small risk of puncturing the liver capsule)
- the upper chest in a grossly cachexic patient (small risk of causing a pneumothorax)
- previously irradiated skin area (within the last eight weeks).

Clinical procedure

The clinical procedure for setting up a syringe driver is based on the North Cumbrian Palliative Care Service Syringe Driver Protocol, with kind permission.

Before starting, explain to the patient and family:

- what the syringe driver is and what it is used for
- why it is needed
- what medication it will contain and what the medication will do
- how to look after the syringe driver
- who to contact if there is concern about malfunction.

Information should be written as well as verbal.

It is important to stress that the syringe driver simply delivers a steady dose of medication by injection. It is not the 'last resort', and in itself can neither shorten nor lengthen life.

Equipment required:

- ✼ Prescription chart and prescribed medication.
- ✼ Syringe driver MS16A or MS26.
- ✼ Protective plastic cover, carrying holster (if appropriate).
- ✼ Two 9-volt batteries.
- ✼ 20 ml syringe with luer lock and needle to draw up drugs.
- ✼ 100 cm Sims Graseby butterfly infusion set (orange needle 25 gauge) or teflon cannula, eg. safe-t-intim.
- ✼ Transparent adhesive dressing, eg. Tegaderm® or iv3000.

⌘ Ampoule of water 10–20 ml for injection.
⌘ Drug additive label for use with syringe drivers.
⌘ Monitoring chart and care plan.

Preparation of medication for administration by syringe driver:

⌘ Calculate the volume of drugs to be given before dilution, then draw up the prescribed drugs and dilute to achieve a total of 48 mm against the mm scale on the front of the syringe driver. When the line is to be primed, draw up 1 ml extra of diluent.
⌘ Connect the syringe to the giving set and prime the line.
⌘ Ensure the label is correctly completed before attaching to the syringe. It is important that the fluid in the barrel of the syringe is visible for measuring purposes.

> The Grasby MS16A (blue front) is set at 02mm/hr = 48 mm over 24 hours
>
> The Graseby MS26 (green front) is set at 48mm/24 hrs = 48 mm over 24 hours

⌘ Check the maintenance date of the syringe driver. If it is more than two months past the maintenance date, do not use and return to the maintenance department. Obtain another syringe driver.
⌘ Ensure the syringe driver to be used is set at the correct rate to enable 48 mm of the drug to be delivered over a twenty-four-hour period.
⌘ Load syringe onto driver and secure.
⌘ Insert battery, press and hold down the 'start' button for five seconds (MS16A) and ten seconds (MS26) and then release to silence the audible alarm and activate the motor. A flashing light will show on the front of the syringe driver to indicate the device is operating.
⌘ Place the driver in the transparent cover and holster if required.
⌘ Ensure the transparent cover is correctly placed with the hole over the 'start' button.

If the total volume exceeds 48 mm on the syringe driver, contact your palliative care team for advice.

Inserting the butterfly infusion set

⌘ Explain the procedure to the patient.
⌘ Assist the patient into a comfortable position.
⌘ Expose the chosen site for infusion.
⌘ Clip excess hair at the site if necessary.
⌘ Grasp the skin firmly, but gently.
⌘ Insert the butterfly needle with the bevel side down at a 45° angle and release grasped skin.
⌘ Tape the infusion wings firmly to the skin using a transparent adhesive dressing.

Continuing care of the patient and the syringe driver

⌘ Ensure that the syringe driver is not placed higher than the infusion site.
⌘ If bolus doses of medication are required, these should be prescribed and given via a separate port or butterfly line ('boosting' does not provide adequate analgesia and leads to premature emptying of the syringe).
⌘ Ensure all initial information is recorded on a monitoring chart.
⌘ Ensure the prescription chart has been signed.
⌘ Check the infusion site and that the volume administered is infusing at the intended rate; record on monitoring chart.
⌘ Monitor any patient symptoms on the care plan.
⌘ The patient should be given a copy of the patient information leaflet and contact numbers in case of problems.
⌘ The site must be changed if there is any redness, swelling, tenderness or leakage.
⌘ If the driver has not gone through on time and there are no other obvious problems with the site or infusion, the syringe driver needs to be examined (see 'Troubleshooting' below).

Troubleshooting

Problems may be:

• with the skin site
• with the syringe driver.

Problems with syringe driver skin sites

From research:

- sites last two to four days (2.35 days in one study, 3–4 days in another).
- skin irritation is perceived as a problem in over one quarter of patients with syringe drivers.
- skin irritation is unrelated to skin site, age, sex, rate of infusion or triceps skin-fold thickness.
- it may relate to diamorphine concentration (one study only); unconfirmed in another study (*Table 7.1*).
- it does seem to be more common with certain drugs. This is anecdotal information.

Table 7.1: Drugs causing skin irritation at syringe driver sites

Rarely cause skin irritation	May cause skin irritation	Too irritant to use
Diamorphine	Levomepromazine (Nozinan)	Chlorpromazine
Metoclopramide	Cyclizine	Prochlorperazine
	Methadone?	
Hyoscine		
Midazolam		

Preventing and controlling skin irritation

Consider:

- changing the site daily
- ensuring the needle is bevel down
- reducing the concentration of irritant drugs
- changing irritant drugs to non-irritant drugs, eg. cyclizine to haloperidol
- giving irritant drugs separately, rectally or intramuscularly (levomepromazine can be given as a single daily injection)
- using saline rather than water as a diluent (the exception is with cyclizine)
- using a small Teflon cannula, such as the safe-t-intima, instead of a butterfly needle
- adding hyaluronidase 1500 units to infusion

- adding dexamethasone to the infusion, in a dose appropriate to the patient's clinical condition. (To add dexamethasone, the diamorphine should be made up with as much water as volume calculation allows. other additions are then made. Dexamethasone is then drawn slowly into the syringe, which is inverted a few times to mix)
- placing a glyceryl trinitrate (GTN) patch over the site of the infusion
- placing the needle intramuscularly rather than subcutaneously.

Problems with the syringe driver (Table 7.2)

Table 7.2: Problems with the syringe driver

Problem	Possible causes	Action
The infusion is too fast (finishing more than an hour early)	• Incorrect rate setting • Scale length measured inaccurately • Use of the 'boost' facility (MS26)	• Check rate setting • Measure scale length carefully • Use bolus doses rather than the 'boost' • Discuss with GP/specialist palliative care team if symptomatic or serious overdose
The infusion is too slow (finishing more than an hour late)	• Incorrect rate setting • Scale length measured inaccurately • Infusion temporarily stopped by patient/family for some reason	• Check rate setting • Measure scale length carefully • Check syringe driver is working (check light is flashing/ battery) • Discuss with GP/specialist palliative care team if unrelieved symptoms or pain
The infusion has stopped	• The battery is exhausted • There is blockage or crystallization in the line • The line is disconnected • The skin site is inflamed	• Replace the battery • Check the syringe/line for crystallization (see below for drug incompatibility problems) • Check the syringe is correctly fitted and the line firmly connected • Change site
The syringe driver will not start	• Battery inserted incorrectly • Battery exhausted • 'Start' button not depressed sufficiently	• Reinsert the battery correctly • Replace the battery • Press the 'start' button firmly for 5 seconds (MS16A) or 10 seconds (MS26)

Discontinuing the syringe driver

When the patient is to receive medication by another route:

- check the alternative medication dose has been accurately calculated from the subcutaneous dose (use 'Approximate opioid equivalents' chart, *Table 2.7.1, p.29* as a guide)
- liaise with the palliative care team, 'drug information' service or on-call pharmacist for advice on timing of alternative route medication
- explain the procedure to the patient
- assist the patient into a comfortable position
- remove battery from syringe driver
- remove giving set, cleanse skin with a mediswab if necessary
- dispose of clear dressing, the giving set and any unused medication in accordance with appropriate trust policies. Dispose of the butterfly following guidelines for the safe disposal of 'sharps'
- return the syringe driver, cover and battery to the collecting point and enter in log book according to local procedure
- the syringe driver should be returned in a clean and ready-to-use condition.

Maintenance of the syringe driver

The outside surfaces of the syringe driver should be cleaned by wiping with a mild detergent in water, and dried. The threads of the screw the actuator moves along can be cleaned using a toothbrush or something similar. Using surgical spirit or other abrasive cleaners may cause damage to the plastic parts. Never dip or immerse the driver in liquid.

Prescribing for the syringe driver

There is **one** indication for using a syringe driver, and that is the patient's inability to take oral medication. The commonest reasons for this are severe dysphagia, vomiting or reduced conscious level. Inadequate pain control indicates a need for pain management review, if necessary seeking additional help or advice. Diazepam, chlorpromazine and prochlorperazine are too irritant to be given subcutaneously.

Which medications should I prescribe? Four groups of drugs are commonly prescribed:

- analgesics (usually diamorphine)
- anti-emetics (haloperidol, cyclizine, metoclopramide, levomepromazine)
- sedatives (midazolam)
- anti-secretory drugs (hyoscine hydrobromide, glycopyrrollate).

Typical doses and indications are listed in *Table 7.3*. Note that:

- a syringe driver takes three to four hours to establish a steady state drug level in plasma. If the patient is in pain, vomiting or agitated, give a single subcutaneous injection of appropriate medication while setting the syringe driver up. Water is the preferred diluent
- the subcutaneous administration of these drugs in various combinations is common practice in palliative care, although this use falls outside the product licence.

Prescriptions are generally written as dose over twenty-four hours. Unless you are prescribing the maximum twenty-four-hour dose in the syringe driver, an additional prescription for bolus doses, as required, through a separate butterfly (with frequency and maximum twenty-four-hour dose) is helpful.

Additional bolus doses of analgesia, as required, should always be prescribed and available for administration by nursing staff when necessary.

What diluent is best to use? Use **water** unless there are problems with site irritation, in which case saline can be used. Never use saline with cyclizine it can cause precipitation.

Can I mix medications in the same syringe? Generally, there are few compatibility problems with common two- and three-drug combinations containing:

- diamorphine
- cyclizine
- haloperidol
- metoclopramide
- levomepromazine
- hyoscine hydrobromide
- midazolam.

Watch out for problems with:

- cyclizine with diamorphine once diamorphine dose exceeds 200 mg/24 hours
- ketorolac (many incompatibilities)
- dexamethasone (common/unpredictable precipitation).

Table 7.3: A brief guide to drugs for the syringe driver

Drug	Dose (subcutaneous)	Comments
Pain		
Diamorphine	If no oral morphine, 10–20 mg/24 hours. Otherwise, total oral morphine given in mg over last 24 hours and divide by 3	Prescribe 1/6 of total 24-hour dose as required for breakthrough pain. Increase 24-hour dose by 1/3 if pain persists
Hyoscine butyl bromide (Buscopan)	60–120 mg/24 hours	Antispasmodic, for bowel or ureteric colic
Vomiting		
Cyclizine	75–150 mg/24 hours. Stable with diamorphine concentrations up to 20 mg/ml (approximates to 200 mg diamorphine/24 hours). May precipitate at higher concentrations*	For vomiting of intestinal obstruction, hepatomegaly or raised intracranial pressure. May cause drowsiness and anticholinergic side-effects
Haloperidol	2.5–10 mg/24 hours	For vomiting caused by opiates (rarely need more than 3 mg/24 hours), uraemia, hypercalcaemia and intestinal obstruction (starting dose 5 mg/24 hours). Non-sedating. Dyskinetic side-effects rare at these doses
Metoclopramide	30–60 mg/24 hours	For vomiting secondary to gastric stasis or gastric compression by ascites, hepatomegaly or intra-abdominal tumour mass
Levomepromazine (methotrimeprazine)	6.25–100 mg/24 hours	Second-line antiemetic for vomiting of intestinal obstruction or in an agitated patient, or where other antiemetics have failed. Sedating at higher doses
Terminal agitation/confusion after excluding untreated pain, full bladder or full rectum		
Haloperidol	5–30 mg/24 hours. Give 5 mg subcutaneously in a single dose while setting up infusion. Can repeat stat dose if needed	Antipsychotic. For confusion with evidence of hallucinations. Risk of dyskinetic side-effects above 10 mg/24 hours. Avoid higher doses if possible
Midazolam	20–100 mg/24 hours. Give 5–10 mg subcutaneously in a single dose while setting up infusion	Water-soluble benzodiazepine. For agitation where there is no evidence of hallucinations. Also used as an anticonvulsant
Hyoscine hydrobromide (scopolamine)	1.6–2.4 mg/24 hours	Sedative, antispasmodic, anti-emetic and reduce secretions
Excess respiratory secretions		
Hyoscine hydrobromide (scopolamine)	1.6–2.4 mg/24 hours	Reduces secretions (give early to prevent build up of secretions). Paradoxical agitation, particularly in the elderly
Glycopyrrollate	0.6–1.2 mg/24 hours	0.2 mg single dose. 2.5 times potency of hyoscine. No central side-effects

Note: The syringe driver takes three to four hours to establish a steady state drug level in plasma. If the patient is in pain, vomiting or very agitated give a stat s/c injection of appropriate medication while setting the syringe driver up. Water is the preferred diluent. The subcutaneous administration of these drugs in various combinations is common practice in palliative care. However, prescribers should be aware that this use falls outside the produce licence. *Dilute diamorphine as much as possible before Cyclizine is added, to avoid concentration dependant crystallization.

Incompatibilty problems can usually be resolved by changing the drugs, giving a drug as a single daily injection or, as a last resort, setting up two syringe drivers (*Table 7.4*).

Table 7.4: Solutions to drug incompatibility problems

Drug	Problem	Solution
Cyclizine	Precipitates with saline and with diamorphine doses >200 mg/24 hours	Use water as diluent. Dilute diamorphine as much as possible before cyclizine is added to avoid concentration depandent crystallisation At higher diamorphine doses, either put cyclizine in a second syringe driver or use levomepromazine as a single, daily, subcutaneous injection instead
Ketorolac	Incompatible with many drugs	Use a separate syringe driver
Dexamethasone	Inactivates glycopyrrollate. Common and unpredictable precipitation with other drugs	Use hyoscine hydrobromide instead of glycopyrrollate. Give dexamethasone as separate, once-daily injection
Hyoscine butyl bromide (Buscopan)	Occasional incompatibility with cyclizine	Give levomepromazine as a single, daily injection in place of cyclizine

Information on compatibility of common two-drug combinations is given in *Figure 7.1*.

More detailed information is available from:

- your local palliative care team
- drug information services
- pharmacists serving specialist inpatient units
- www.palliativedrugs.com
- www.pallmed.net

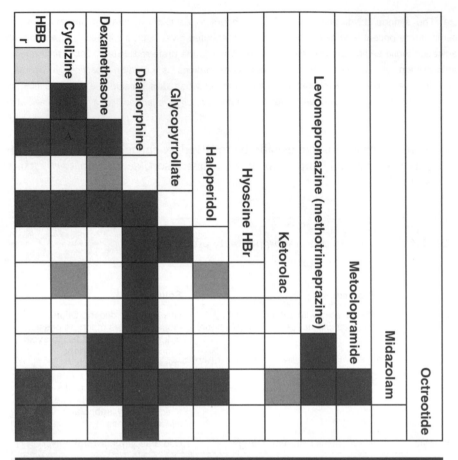

A brief guide to syringe driver compatibility for two drugs

Incompatible (lab or PCU data)

Sometimes incompatible (PCU data)

Compatible (lab or PCU data)

No data available

Figure 7.1: Compatibility of common two-drug combinations

Key points

❖ Syringe drivers have helped transform delivery of palliative care in the home setting, and skill in their use is vital.

❖ The syringe driver may be used in any situation when the patient is unable to take oral medication.

❖ A syringe driver is only an alternative method of administering medication. It does not produce more effective analgesia than the oral route unless the patient cannot use oral medication or has serious compliance problems, nor should it be routinely used as a 'medical last rite'.

❖ Where local guidelines or protocols are available, the primary care team should access and follow them.

❖ Syringe drivers should only be set up by staff trained and competent in their use.

❖ Different types of syringe driver are used in different areas. This often causes confusion, and sometimes serious hazard when staff move from one area to another.

❖ It is vitally important to check the model of syringe driver you are using, to ensure you are familiar with it and to follow the manufacturer's guidelines for that model carefully.

❖ Syringe driver prescriptions are written as the total dose/24 hours. As necessary bolus doses may still be required, especially for painkillers.

❖ The prescriber should be aware of potential drug incompatibilities, and know where to access detailed information.

Further reading — syringe drivers

Department of Health (1994) *Doing No Harm*. The Medical Devices Directorate, Department of Health, London

Department of Health (1995) *The Report of the Expert Working Group on Alarms and Clinical Monitors*. The Medical Devices Directorate, Department of Health, London

Fallon M, O'Neill B (1998) *ABC of Palliative Care*. BMJ Books, London

Graseby (1998) *MS16A and MS26 Instruction Manual*. SIMS

Kaye P (1994) *A–Z Pocketbook of Symptom Control*. EPL Publications, Oxford

North Cumbria Palliative Care Service Syringe Driver Protocol. Available online at: www.northcumbriahealth.nhs.uk/palliative care

Oliver DJ (1988) Syringe drivers in palliative care: a review. *Palliative Med* **2**: 21–6

Regnard C, Tempest S (1998) *A Guide to Symptom Relief in Advanced Cancer*. 4th edn. Radcliffe Medical Press, Oxford

Twycross R, Wilcock A (2001) *Symptom Management in Advanced Cancer.* 3rd edn. Radcliffe Medical Press, Oxford

Twycross R, Wilcock A, Thorp S (2002) *Palliative Care Formulary.* 2nd edn. Radcliffe Medical Press, Oxford

Syringe driver manual

Setting the rate

It is essential the operator identifies the model of syringe driver being used and understands the difference between the two models.

MS16A (blue cover)

Hourly rate, ie. rate is in millimetres of syringe plunger travel per one hour.

MS16A   Rate =

$$\text{Rate} = \frac{\text{Measured 'length of volume' in mm}}{\text{Delivery time in hours}}$$

eg.

$$\frac{48 \text{ mm}}{24h} = 2mm/h$$

MS26 (green cover)

Daily rate, ie. rate is in millimetres of syringe plunger travel per 24 hours.

MS26   Rate =

$$\text{Rate} = \frac{\text{Measured 'length of volume' in mm}}{\text{Delivery time in days}}$$

eg.

$$\frac{48}{1} = 48mm/24h$$

Length of volume

Preparing the syringe driver

Step 1 : Prepare the syringe

❖   Use a luer lock 20ml syringe

❖   Using the 'mm' measuring scale on the side of the syringe driver (Diagram 2) measure the number of millilitres (mls) in your syringe equivalent to the length of 48mm. Always measure from zero on the syringe scale up to the line where the plunger piston is. This is your volume (Diagram 1).

❖ Draw up the prescribed medication to the correct volume.

❖ If using a new infusion line (ie. on initial setting up or when resiting the infusion) draw up an additional 1 ml of diluent. This is the correct additional volume required to fill the line using the Graseby 100cm infusion set as recommended.

❖ Complete the details on a yellow drug label and attach to syringe. Do not obscure the syringe scale.

Step 2 : Connect the infusion set to the syringe

❖ Use a 100 cm Graseby Infusion Set.

❖ Connect it securely to the syringe.

❖ If it is a new infusion set gently depress the syringe plunger until the line is just full (1 ml volume).

Step 3 : Prepare the syringe driver

❖ Check the model of syringe driver: MS16 (BLUE — rate is in mm/1hr) or MS26 (GREEN — rate is in mm/24hrs).

❖ Set the correct rate (see page 1) DOUBLE CHECK.

❖ Install the battery. The alarm should sound.

Step 4 : Start the syringe driver

❖ Press and hold down the start button. The motor will turn and stop after 5 secs (MS16) or 10 secs (MS26). Then the alarm will sound. This checks the syringe driver safety system. If the motor fails to stop or the alarm does not sound, do not use the syringe driver.

❖ Once the 'start' button is released the indicator lamp will flash (Diagram 2) (MS16 every 1 sec) or (MS26 every 25 secs). The syringe driver is now running. If the lamp does not flash, try replacing the battery.

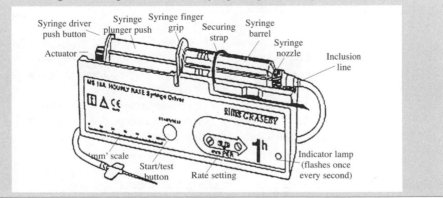

Step 5 : Fitting the syringe to the syringe driver

❖ Place the syringe on top of the driver so that the syringe finger grip fits into the slot in the syringe driver case (Diagrams 2 and 3).

❖ Secure the syringe firmly with the rubber strap (Diagrams 2 and 3).

❖ Press the white square button (Diagram 4). You can now slide the actuator gently towards the syringe plunger button (Diagram 2) until the end of the syringe plunger sits firmly in the slot of the actuator (Diagram 4).

❖ Place syringe driver in clear plastic cover. The hole must be over the start button.

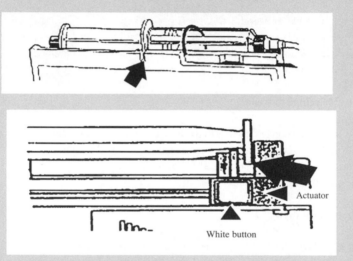

Step 6 : Connect the infusion set to the patient

❖ Insert the needle inverted (ie. bevel down) at an angle of 30–45° into subcutaneous tissue at an appropriate site.

❖ Secure the needle with a transparent dressing. Include a loop of the infusion set under the dressing to avoid any direct pull on the needle.

❖ Ensure patient and carers know that the syringe driver must NOT be placed at a level higher than the infusion site (it is possible for the contents to syphon out).

❖ If you are still unsure of the procedure or have any other questions please refer to either the SIMS GRASEBY Syringe Driver Instruction Manual or the North Cumbria Palliative Care Service Syringe Driver Protocol.

❖ If you are still in doubt do not proceed and seek advice.

Part 2
Psychological

8

Breaking bad news — loss and adjustment reactions

8.1 What is bad news?

Bad news is news that implies loss of something that the person values and is attached to.

Bad news is information that causes the person receiving it to re-evaluate a basic expectation in an unwanted way. Information alone is neither good nor bad. Its impact depends on the individual — his or her ideas, expectations, age, personality, approach to life, social situation and so on. This is an important concept. It explains why one person might be devastated by a relatively innocuous diagnosis, having never prepared him or herself for anything other than perfect health, and maybe having ambitious life plans. Another person might take a serious diagnosis with a short prognosis completely in his or her stride, having a deep lifelong acceptance of death as a natural stage of his or her life, with no negative connotations. These are extreme examples. However, many doctors and nurses will meet patients who cope well with the diagnosis, but are then devastated by a treatment side-effect that means they cannot work. Someone else who has battled with progressive disability for years may find news of a limited life expectancy 'good'.

8.2 Loss

Loss is a gap between expectation, belief, desire and reality. Loss can be:

- loss of physical health

- loss of expectation of physical health in the future
- loss of emotional wellbeing or peace of mind
- loss of social functions, such as roles at work, within the family, independence in self-care, body and self-image
- loss of social expectations, such as seeing children/grandchildren through life's milestones, to maintain an income, to finish a project, to develop a hobby or interest, to travel
- loss of spiritual sustenance, such as disconnection, abandonment, loss of meaning, impending loss of important relationships, questioning or loss of belief system.

There is more about loss in *Chapter 23: Grief, mourning and bereavement.*

It is said that the whole of human existence can be thought of as a series of losses of varying degrees, from when the warmth and stability of intra-uterine life comes to an abrupt end at birth! A serious illness such as cancer involves facing a whole series of losses. There may be little time to adjust to one loss, before the next loss comes. Each loss also has the power to touch on and reactivate feelings and memories from previous losses. It is common for patients to describe powerful memories of a parent's death, or a friend's experience with cancer.

These memories and feelings impact on the patient's experience and expectations. Human beings have psychological mechanisms designed to help them to cope with loss and with bad news; this is vital for psychological survival. Loss precipitates what is called an adjustment reaction, which allows the person to assimilate the loss and come to a new point of psychological stability. These sorts of reactions proceed on many levels, and a deeper understanding is given in *Chapter 19: Holistic care and the cancer journey* (19.2. The experience of a serious illness as a journey) and in *Chapter 22: Spiritual care in a secular society* (22.5. What is spiritual pain?).

8.3 The 'normal' adjustment reaction

It is important to remember that it is normal to react emotionally to bad news.

Initial reactions

Common initial reactions are:

- denial — 'I don't believe it'

- numbness — 'I'm shocked, I feel like it's not happening'
- anger — 'If only they had done the tests sooner'
- grief, with tears and sadness.

These reactions depend on the size of the loss and the usual coping mechanisms of the person. Sometimes there is visible anxiety and fear.

Many people are skilled at 'keeping a brave face on things' and may conduct a rational dialogue, while many thoughts, fears and feelings are racing through their mind. It is little wonder that later recall of detail given after the 'bad news' is incomplete and inaccurate.

Early reactions

There may be anger, guilt, anxiety and sadness. There may be a need for further information, and a re-checking of information already given. This is partly because of the incomplete hearing of information described above; it is also a way of re-confirming the reality of the situation as the mind struggles to come to terms with it.

There is often a need to tell and re-tell the story. Previous experience and memory re-surfaces, and may contribute positively or negatively to the patient's hopes and fears. Anger may be expressed towards other family members as rage or irritability. It is also frequently directed towards members of the healthcare teams, and the hospital or the GP may be blamed for real or perceived failings in diagnosis or treatment.

Inner 'bargaining' is common, such as 'I'll do anything, anything at all if only this can get better again'. Normal coping can vary from taking a detailed interest in treatments and new advances from all over the world, to leaving everything in the 'experts' hands.

Later reactions and coping mechanisms

Eventually, after a period of days to weeks, longer-term coping strategies emerge. Four are commonly described:

- fighting spirit ('I will not let this beat me')
- stoical acceptance ('I have got it, I will get on with it')
- denial ('There is nothing wrong with me')
- resigned helplessness ('What's the point, I cannot make a difference').

There have been suggestions that those who cope using a 'fighting spirit' or by denial might survive longer, although the evidence for this has been challenged (see also 'different coping mechanisms in the family'). Even after being carefully informed that there was no expectation of cure from palliative radiotherapy for advanced cancer, 58% of patients still expected to recover. These patients experienced a significantly better quality of life than those who believed the only benefit would be pain control.

It is quite normal for patients to ask the same questions several times, perhaps to different professionals, as part of their gradual assimilation of the loss associated with a terminal diagnosis. Most of us find some coping styles easier to deal with than others, and it is helpful to have some personal insight into this.

8.4 Breaking bad news

Most patients with cancer want to know their diagnosis. Most doctors want to tell patients their diagnosis. Despite this, giving bad news remains one of the greatest challenges of the doctor's work.

The primary care physician is usually involved. There are some common and consistent behaviours that can make a big difference:

- finding a quiet place for the consultation
- having enough time, avoiding interruptions
- the conversation being face to face
- giving some warning, such as 'I am afraid the news is not good'
- the conversation proceeding at the patient's pace (giving time for it to 'sink in')
- a sense for the patient of being listened to
- the sense that support is available.

There is a small but significant subgroup of patients who do not wish to know their diagnosis (about 10%). In terms of content and level of detail, most patients want to know that the diagnosis is cancer. Fewer want to know the exact medical name of their illness (30%). Fewer still want to know the prognosis (which is difficult to give with honesty and certainty except in general terms). However, almost all want to know the chance of a cure. The worse the prognosis, the less patients want to know.

Few people find breaking bad news easy, but it is possible to become more skilful at it. While this cannot alter the news itself, it can go some way to reduce the chances of overwhelming patients too quickly, so they go into total denial or panic. What patients and families remember most later will be the kindness with which it was done. Most doctors do care about their patients at times like this. Showing this by word or gesture can make all the difference.

He was only a young doctor. He didn't seem to know what to say, but he had tears in his eyes. I knew he really cared about her, about us.

The doctor came to say they had found seedlings in his liver. Then when I saw a CAT scan of that, it was a huge tumour that had gone right through his liver. The pain in his shoulder was cancer in the bones. You know it was pretty horrible. I was in such a frozen state of panic in my own mind, thinking 'How am I going to cope with all this, how is he going to cope with this?' that I didn't really consider what they said. But I do remember they were very gentle and very tactful, and they were extremely nice to him.

There are several strategies for breaking bad news. If the patient or family are totally unprepared, it is a big psychological transition. Whatever strategy you use, it is helpful to remember the following key points.

Before you start

Have you got the information you need? Is it accurate and up-to date? Have you got a planned safety net in case the patient needs a quiet space and listening ear at the end of the consultation? (For example, the patient is arriving with a close family member/friend; the nurse is available and knows we are going to discuss this.)

Breaking bad news: Step 1 — Find out what is already known:

⌘   What have the patient/family been told?
⌘   What have they understood by this?
⌘   What do they make of it themselves? (This may be very different from what they have been told!)
⌘   This establishes the starting point. Often patients and families have guessed the diagnosis; you can then gently confirm it, check their feelings and concerns (see Step 5, below) and carry on from there.
⌘   If they have no idea, you need to warn them that bad news is coming.

This step also allows you to check the words they use and what they understand from them.

Patient: *He said I had a tumour that had spread, but not to worry because he is going to do an operation.*
GP: *So what do you understand by that?*

Patient: *Well, at least it's not cancer.*

I was given an X-ray form that had written on it 'To rule out metastases'. No-one had mentioned cancer yet, and no-one had checked I was a nurse.

Breaking bad news: Step 2 — Give warning that bad news is coming:

I am afraid it looks like something more serious than that...   or

I have some bad news for you.

If the patient has used specific words, start by using these words:

It is something more serious than a simple ulcer.   or

You have got a tumour, but it is more serious than that.

This is done with careful attention and sensitivity to the patient's response. It gives a position of real choice to the patient (*Figure 8.4.1*).

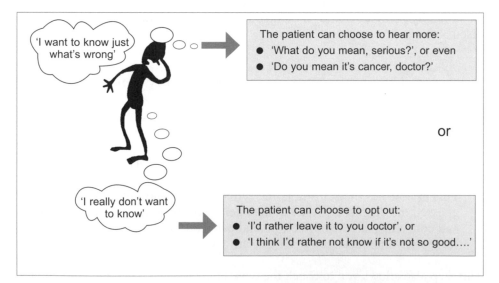

Figure 8.4.1: Giving the patient warning that bad news is coming gives a position of choice to the patient

⌘   Do not give information if the patient asks you not to. Respect his or her choice, and leave an opening for further discussion: 'That's fine. Would it be OK if I just check with you from time to time how you are and if you need any more information about your illness?'

⌘   Allow denial, again leaving an opening for further discussion if wanted.

Breaking bad news: Step 3 — Give information in 'bite-size' chunks:

⌘   Break the information down into gradated steps. This slows and paces the consultation, giving the patient space and time to take it in.

⌘   If giving a serious diagnosis, a 'hierarchy of euphemisms' can be useful — 'abnormal cells', 'looks malignant', 'it is cancer'.

⌘   Keep information clear, simple and jargon-free.

⌘   Repeat the main points — mini summaries are useful.

⌘   Keep the choice of words kind and positive. Words and phrases such as 'incurable cancer', 'terminal cancer', and 'there is nothing more we can do' or 'you are going to die' are harsh, and should be avoided. They can precipitate helplessness and panic, leading people to lose all hope.

⌘   A simple, clear message is what is needed — 'This is a cancer in the lung' or 'the cancer has come back in the thigh bone, close to the hip'.

⌘   Avoid giving too much complex, medical information at this point unless directly asked.

Breaking bad news: Step 4 — Wait for it all to sink in:

⌘   It can feel such a relief to have said the 'hard bits' that there is a great temptation to carry on with the rest of the consultation.

⌘   The patient is meanwhile making a big transition and may not be able to keep up with you.

⌘   Be sensitive — look and listen for verbal and non-verbal clues to how the patient is feeling.

Breaking bad news: Step 5 — Check how they feel and if they have any questions:

⌘   If there is visible distress, notice and acknowledge it — 'I can see that's been a bit of a shock' or 'That has upset you…'

⌘   Otherwise ask specifically about feelings, fears, concerns and questions — 'How does that leave you feeling?'

⌘   The doctor's role here is to listen; do not try to solve it all (and do not assume you know the patient's real concerns — the patient is usually the best judge of that).

Following diagnosis it was suggested, demanded really, that I should have lots of questions, and most particularly the question 'Why me?' Without waiting, the doctor proceeded to answer that question for me by telling me there was no answer. I actually had no such question! Why not me? Me as much as anyone else. I don't recall we ever got to questions that were mine.

Patient with newly diagnosed cancer.

Check you have all the patients concerns:

Is anything else bothering you?   or

Are there any other questions?

Check the patient understands what you have said.

Breaking bad news: Step 6 — Agree a plan

⌘ Don't leave things up in the air — agree a clear plan for the way forward.
⌘ Summarize and prioritize concerns with the patient.
⌘ Focus on things that can be done.
⌘ Balance realism with the importance of realistic hope — 'We cannot always cure cancer, but we may be able to slow it down', 'We can definitely help to get things easier for you than they are right now' or 'Prepare for the worst, but hope for the best'.
⌘ Do not rush the patient into complex treatment decisions.
⌘ Check strategy for informing key family members. Does the patient want to do this? Would they like you to do this?
⌘ Give a safety net, such as a review date and explain what the patient should do or who to call if there are concerns before that date.
⌘ If the patient has brought a close family member, remember information needs and pace may differ, sometimes significantly. Keep the focus on the patient, but offer to see the family member separately if necessary.

Patient: *One week later we were told it was terminal. In my naïve state of mind, I thought if you can't cure it maybe they could make it so you could live with it. So they laid it on us — no, it was terminal. Neither of us had the courage to ask how long; it was too scary.*

Doctor: *Would you have wanted to know?*

Patient: *No, not really.*

8.5 Providing supportive care for normal adjustment

There is some evidence that good psychosocial support (including support groups) may assist the process of normal adjustment. As the information is assimilated, many patients value a friendly professional with listening skills. Listening is probably the most important skill at this stage. Patients may ask difficult questions, sometimes of a relatively unexpected or inexperienced team member. These questions take a lot of courage to ask, and they should always be heard and acknowledged, even if it is not possible to give an answer. It is also important to clarify **what** the person is asking and **why** they are asking it just now. It is easy to make assumptions that are wrong.

Example

A very ill man asked the nurse 'What happens to people after they die?' She took a deep breath and gave a long explanation of many belief systems, ranging from reincarnation to a 'simple sleep and a forgetting'. He listened with interest, then said 'I was thinking more about the wife, and maybe getting in touch with an undertaker, and that sort of thing.'

If asked a difficult question:

⌘   Always indicate you have heard the question.
⌘   Take a few minutes to check just what it is the patient wants to know and why.
⌘   Check they do want an answer. Many difficult questions are asked to open a dialogue. 'Answers' quickly and effectively close dialogue.
⌘   Most difficult questions are difficult because they do not have an answer that is certain.
⌘   Be honest if you do not know. If appropriate, offer to find out or to arrange for a consultation with someone who may be better placed to deal with the question.
⌘   Acknowledge the difficulty of uncertainty.

It is often hard to say 'I don't know'. Both professional credibility and pressure from patients and families can make us feel we should give an answer. Untrue answers, such as 'He has six months at the most' or 'The hospital will cure it', cause far more distress for patients and families, and rebound badly on your professional credibility.

8.6 Talking about dying

Elizabeth Kübler-Ross (1970) worked extensively with people who were facing death. Her book *On Death and Dying* described the stages she observed people go through in their attitude as they came nearer to death. They closely mirror the adjustment reaction described above. They are:

- denial — 'This cannot possibly be happening to me'
- anger — 'Why me?'
- bargaining — 'I will never smoke again if I can just live long enough to see my grandchild'
- depression, grief, mourning, sadness and despair
- acceptance — a letting go and quiet resignation to the impending death. (This stage is not inevitable, but where it occurs it is accompanied by a sense of peace and often a withdrawal, a wish to be quiet. The struggle is over.)

This sort of model can be helpful, but it is only a model. Human beings rarely travel through their emotions in such a neat and orderly fashion. In reality, all of these stages can be experienced in different parts of the same day. Patients may be peaceful and accepting one day, and angry the next.

However, it conveys the sense of an underlying journey, which is explored more in *Chapter 19: Holistic care and the cancer journey*.

One of Dr Kübler-Ross's observations was that once patients had accepted and were able to talk about their impending death, they often died soon after. We must not expect patients to want to talk extensively about their dying until they are ready to do so. We should be willing to leave the door open for the patient to talk about dying when they are ready.

Recognizing poor adjustment and mood disorders

There are some features that may predict a poor adjustment. These include:

- a negative appraisal of information

- a large number of concerns
- concerns that do not resolve
- past psychiatric history
- low self-esteem
- a coping style of helplessness.

Poor adjustment may result in anxiety disorders, fear or terror. One-quarter of patients with cancer develop clinical depression.

Key points

❖ Bad news is news that implies loss of something that the person values and is attached to.

❖ Most patients with cancer want to know their diagnosis. Most doctors want to tell patients their diagnosis. Despite this, giving bad news remains one of the greatest challenges of doctors' work.

❖ Few people find breaking bad news easy, but it is possible to become more skillful at it.

❖ What patients and families remember most later will be the kindness with which it was done. Most doctors do care about their patients at times like this. Showing this by word or gesture can make all the difference.

❖ It is normal to react emotionally to bad news.

❖ Most difficult questions are difficult because they do not have an answer that is certain. Be honest if you do not know, and acknowledge the difficulty of uncertainty.

❖ Many difficult questions are asked to open a dialogue. 'Answers' quickly and effectively close dialogue.

Further reading

Buckman R (1988) *I Don't Know What to Say. How to Help and Support Someone who is Dying*. Macmillan Medical, London

Buckman R (1993) *How to Break Bad News. A Guide for Healthcare Professionals*. Macmillan Medical, London

Buckman R (1994) Breaking bad news: why is it so difficult? *Br Med J* **288**: 1597–9

Faulkner A, Maguire P (1988a) How to do it: improve the counselling skills of doctors and nurses in cancer care. *Br Med J* **297**: 847–9

Faulkner A, Maguire P (1988b) How to do it: communicate with cancer patients 1. Handling bad news and difficult questions. *Br Med J* **297**: 907–9

Faulkner A, Maguire P (1994) *Talking to Cancer Patients and their Relatives*. Oxford Medical Publications, Oxford

Franks A (1997) Breaking bad news and the challenge of communication. *Eur J Palliative Care* **4**: 61–4

Hogbin *et al* (1992) Remembering bad news consultations: an evaluation of tape-recorded consultations. *Psycho-oncology* **1**: 147–54

Kaye P (1996) *Breaking Bad News: a Ten-Step Approach*. EPL Publications, Northampton

Kübler-Ross E (1970) *On Death and Dying*. Tavistock, London

Meredith C, Symonds P, Webster L *et al* (1996) Information needs of cancer patients in West Scotland: cross-sectional survey of patients' views. *Br Med J* **313**: 724–6

Siverman J, Kurtz S, Draper J (1998) *Skills for Communicating with Patients*. Radcliffe Medical Press, Oxford

Stedeford A (1984) *Facing Death*. Heinemann, London

9

Anxiety

Anxiety is common. It ranges from mild and fleeting to severe and disabling.

9.1 Common clinical situations

Specific (situational) anxiety

This is anxiety around specific situations, such as injections, chemotherapy and hospital appointments. Consider appropriate interventions, such as:

- topical local anaesthetic (EMLA) cream
- the company of a friend or trusted health worker
- talking through and preparing questions and strategies for likely situations
- short-acting benzodiazepines, such as lorazepam 1–2mg, to cover the event
- mental training with hypnotherapy, relaxation training or meditation.

Generalized anxiety

Exclude a depressive illness (see *Chapter 11: Depression*). Check whether this is a new symptom or part of a lifelong personality pattern, and adjust your treatment goals accordingly.

9.2 Tackling the out-of-control feeling

Anxiety often relates to feeling out of control, and measures that give the patient a sense of control can be helpful:

- giving clear information about the illness and the reason for symptoms
- sharing treatment decisions
- sharing the care plan so the patient can know what to expect, who does what and also how and when to contact key individuals
- giving the patient choices wherever possible
- respecting these choices
- respecting a patient's wish to leave decision making 'to the professionals'.

A skilled family doctor or district nurse may be able to encourage the anxious patient to disclose his or her worries and fears, and where possible work out strategies to deal with them. Patients do not always like to use words such as 'worry' or 'fear', thinking that this may reflect poorly on their coping skills. Asking whether they have any concerns or questions about how things are going may be more effective.

Some practices may bring in the practice counsellor or have rapid access to psychology services. Relaxation training, cognitive behaviour therapy and hypnotherapy may be useful. Some anxious patients find it difficult to talk, but may respond to touch therapies such as massage, aromatherapy or Reiki. Others (often, but not always men) may deal with anxiety through practical activity; 'DIY', woodwork, walking and gardening are common outlets. Drug treatment for generalized anxiety is with benzodiazepines. Lorazepam 1–2 mg twice-daily is suitable. If there is sleep disturbance, diazepam 2–10 mg at night may be preferred.

9.3 Anxiety with panic attacks

Explanation and behavioural techniques, such as breathing slowly while counting, can sometimes enable patients to control their panic attacks. If attacks are infrequent, lorazepam 0.5–2 mg administered sublingually at the start of an attack can bring rapid relief. The mouth is often dry during a panic attack. It is worth explaining this to the patient and suggesting they take a small sip of water to swill around the mouth before using sublingual lorazepam. For frequent and severe attacks, paroxetine 20 mg daily is licensed for panic disorder. The general approaches to anxiety above are also worth trying.

10

Fear and terror

Fear and terror usually relate to deep existential and spiritual distress. This has been referred to as 'soul pain'. It is dealt with in more detail in Part 4. This is usually distressing for the whole team, who may feel powerless.

Key points in the management of fear and terror

⌘ Deep fear and terror is one of the hardest things for a team to manage.
⌘ Acknowledge that and support each other.
⌘ It is also distressing and frightening for families who may need 'permission' for respite.
⌘ A quiet, steady, listening presence, 'listening with the heart and soul', cannot be underestimated.
⌘ Check the patient's orientation and understanding — is this an early confusional state?
⌘ Check for depression
⌘ Try to explore illness belief systems and beliefs around death and dying.
⌘ Are there important spiritual beliefs that might mean comfort from a priest or religious leader would help?
⌘ What sort of things have helped and sustained the patient in previous life crises?
~ does he/she love music?
~ a special friend?
~ a favourite passage from a book or piece of poetry?
~ the sound of running water or the scent of roses?
This may give family members a sense of meaningful and calmer ways to support their fearful relative.
⌘ Use a multidisciplinary approach, including family, spiritual support, psychology, social work, creative and diversional therapies where appropriate.
⌘ Involve specialist services early to support team, patient and family.

⌘ Consider complementary therapies. Fear and terror that the patient cannot talk through can sometimes respond well to touch therapies. Massage, aromatherapy and Reiki can be used.

⌘ Consider drug side-effects. Terror can sometimes occur as an idiosyncratic reaction to haloperidol or to too much opioid. It can also respond to major tranquillizers or benzodiazepines (which may need to be given in substantial doses).

⌘ Resistant fear and terror can sometimes respond to paroxetine 20 mg daily or clonazepam 0.5–2 mg daily (the latter is cumulative so the dose will need reducing over time).

11

Depression

Most patients will experience sadness. About 50% of patients will experience a symptomatic adjustment reaction, with sadness, anger, grief, anxiety and fear. This will gradually resolve over a number of weeks or months with the patient's own resources, and support from family, friends and health professionals.

The resolution of an adjustment reaction can be recognized by:

- active involvement in normal life activities
- minimal disruption to usual roles (partner, parent, worker, etc)
- ability to manage the normal emotional impact of illness
- ability to manage difficult feelings, ie. guilt, powerlessness and helplessness.

Up to one-quarter of patients with cancer will develop clinical depression. Half of these are neither diagnosed nor treated. Patients and families can wrongly assume depression to be inevitable or unavoidable. Doctors and nurses can share this view, or be too focused on physical aspects of care to notice or ask. Yet depression, like fatigue and existential or spiritual distress, can impact severely on overall quality of life.

Depression in palliative care: Step 1 — suspect depression

Specific risk factors include:

- previous depression
- a weak social support system (single or living alone, lack of local family/ friends, isolated work environment)
- a serious prognosis
- marked functional disability from cancer
- persistent negative ideas and beliefs
- recent bereavement
- pancreatic cancer.

Remember, however, that any patient can develop depression.

Depression in palliative care: Step 2 — diagnose

⌘ A single screening question, such as 'Are you depressed?', provides sensitive and specific assessment.

⌘ Core diagnostic features are:
  ~ pervasive low mood and/or
  ~ loss of interest or pleasure in anything lasting at least two weeks.

⌘ Grief and adjustment reactions tend to fluctuate; depression is constant and unremitting.

⌘ Physical symptoms are much less reliable in diagnosing depression in palliative care patients, who may have disturbance in appetite, weight loss and fatigue as cancer-related symptoms.

⌘ Psychological symptoms are much more reliable. Hopelessness, helplessness, worthlessness, guilt, social withdrawal and suicidal thoughts all add to the likelihood of clinical depression.

Depression in palliative care: Step 3 — treat

⌘ Have a low threshold for treating depression in the terminally ill.
⌘ Control pain.
⌘ Supportive therapy/counselling (if depression is severe, this may need to be postponed until antidepressant therapy is working).
⌘ Refer to the community specialist psychiatric care team or day hospice/ palliative care team.
⌘ Prescribe an antidepressant.

Choice of drugs

Tricyclic antidepressants:

• amitriptyline 25–150 mg daily
• dothiepin 25–150 mg daily
• venlafaxine 37.5–75 mg twice-daily (may be regarded as an amitriptyline-like drug with fewer side-effects).

These drugs should improve sleep within days, stimulate the appetite and weight gain. The co-analgesic effect is usually within three to seven days. The antidepressant effect may take two to four weeks.

Selective serotonin reuptake inhibitors (SSRIs). For example, paroxetine 20 mg once-daily. Also licensed for anxiety and panic disorder. May take up to four weeks to exert antidepressant effect. No recognized co-analgesic effect.

Psychostimulants. One US consensus recommends these as drugs of choice for depressed patients with a short prognosis. For example, methylphenidate 5 mg twice-daily gradually titrated up to 10 or 15 mg twice-daily. Response is within days, but one-third will experience side-effects.

Hypericum (St John's Wort). Popular and well-tolerated herbal remedy widely available without prescription. As effective as tricyclics for mild/moderate depression, with fewer side-effects. Problems can arise from hepatic enzyme induction, drug interactions and lack of standardization between different formulations. Important interactions are listed in the back of the *British National Formulary* under 'St John's Wort'.

If the patient is not responding, consider early referral to a community psychiatric team, a psycho-oncology service, or a specialist palliative care service for advice and assessment.

12

Insomnia

Managing insomnia in palliative care: Step 1 — is there a correctable cause?

⌘   Is pain and symptom control adequate?
⌘   Does the patient have unresolved concerns or fears (see *Chapters 9* and *10*)?
⌘   Is the sleeping environment satisfactory?
⌘   Has depression been excluded (see *Chapter 11*)?
⌘   Is medication contributing (*Table 12.1*)?

Table 12.1: Effects of drugs on insomnia

Drug	Effect on sleep	Reduce by
Opioids	Commonly improve sleep quality if pain is a problem Nightmares if dose too high	Dose adjustment Add in co-analgesic Try a different opioid
Corticosteroids	Mildly stimulating if given late in the day	Give as single morning dose or twice-daily dose with last dose at lunchtime
Caffeine/theophyllines	Central nervous system stimulants	Restrict use to early in the day or try without
Alcohol	Small amounts may improve sleep; larger amounts commonly produce insomnia	Reduce intake/ try without
Diuretics	Nocturia	Use shorter-acting agents, earlier in the day
Bronchodilators	Central nervous system stimulants	Reduce dose if possible Use inhaled rather than oral formulations

Managing insomnia in palliative care: Step 2 — general sleep hygiene:

⌘ Attention to the environment: quiet, comfortable, dark.
⌘ Good sleep/wake cycle. Reduce cat-napping if excessive.
⌘ Physical activity where possible.
⌘ Quiet and relaxing evening activities.
⌘ Relaxation tapes/calming music.
⌘ Massage/aromatherapy.

Managing insomnia in palliative care: Step 3 — consider prescribing:

⌘ Night sedation, such as temazepam 10–40 mg at night.
⌘ Antidepressants if depressed or early-morning waking, such as amitriptyline 25 mg at night.
⌘ A sedating antihistamine if pruritis is a cause, such as promethazine 25–50 mg at night.
⌘ Levomepromazine 12.5–50 mg at night (this can be very sedating; start low, build up slowly).

13

Confusion and agitation

Confusion and agitation can be immensely distressing and frightening symptoms, particularly for the family, but also for the patient if there is insight. They present a challenge for the primary care team to manage at home.

13.1 Confusion and pseudoconfusion

It is helpful to be clear about terminology. 'Confusion' is usually defined as a global defect in cognition. 'Pseudoconfusion' may arise from disordered sensory input, for example from deafness, anxiety or being too ill to concentrate. Verbal expression may be muddled because of expressive dysphasia or concentration defects.

True confusion is secondary to a defect in cerebral processing. This is commonly divided into delirium (an acute, intermittent and potentially reversible situation caused by a noxious insult to the brain) and dementia (a chronic, progressive and irreversible situation caused by brain damage). A patient with dementia may have an exacerbation of their chronic confusion by an acute organic cause; likewise, a patient with an organic delirium may have a degree of underlying dementia exposed.

13.2 Delirium and dementia

Both delirium and dementia share some common features:

- short-term memory impairment
- disorientation — time, place, person
- concentration reduced
- misinterpretations

- delusions
- hallucinations.

The clinical features listed in *Table 13.2.1* help differentiate them.

Table 13.2.1: Key clinical features differentiating delirium and dementia

Feature to ask about	Delirium	Dementia
• When did it start?	Acute onset	Chronic
• Does it come and go?	May be variable/reversible	Progressive/irreversible
• Is the patient more sleepy than usual?	Drowsy (mental clouding)	Not drowsy
• Is there a difference through the 24 hours?	Diurnal variation	Constant
• Does the patient seem aware they are sometimes mixed up/forgetful?	Insight and anxiety	Lack of insight/concern

---

13.3 The sensory filter model

We are all continuously bombarded with sensory input from the body, the unconscious mind and the environment. This model postulates that to function in an effective and focused way a filter blocks much of this sensory input for most of the time so our attention is not distracted unnecessarily. Confusion occurs when this filter ceases to function effectively. The confused patient is overwhelmed by usually filtered sensory input; the ability to localize the source of the input is lost, so misinterpretations are common. For example, pyrexia may be perceived as the room on fire; subconscious fears may lead to the perception of unfamiliar faces as dangerous; memories from long ago may be perceived as current events.

13.4 Managing confusion

Managing confusion in palliative care: Step 1 — general management:

- ⌘ **Explanation.** Explanation to patient, family and professional colleagues is vital. Lay people fear the patient is going mad or losing his or her mind. Carers feel they have lost the vital part of the person they love; this is much harder to bear than many physical symptoms. Explanation that this is not madness, that it is probably multifactorial, and the sense of a calm and professional management plan that engages the carers as full partners will optimize the chances of managing this difficult situation well.
- ⌘ **Environment.** Decide the care setting with the family and patient, assessing the amount of lay and professional support necessary and the degree of supervision the patient needs. Gentle lighting, familiar faces, a familiar care setting if possible and a small number of staff help to reduce the potential for exacerbation of the confusion. Safety needs to be addressed. A mattress on the floor may be safer than cot sides. Hazards such as stairs, matches, medication, doors opening into busy roads and gas fires need talking through with lay carers.
- ⌘ **Calming influences.** A calm, professional manner inspires confidence. Soothing music may help, as may familiar, repetitive rituals, such as washing or brushing the patient's hair. Verbal reorientation is often helpful: 'I am Dr Jones. It's Tuesday today and it's cold outside. It's December and it will soon be Christmas'.

Managing confusion in palliative care: Step 2 — correct the correctable

Common causes are:

- infection — usually chest or urine
- drugs — opioids, psychotropics, steroids
- drug withdrawal — opioids, nicotine, alcohol
- hypoxia
- dehydration
- raised intracranial pressure
- hypercalcaemia
- retention of urine, constipation, pain.

Provided the patient is not in the last few days of life, baseline assessment and investigation should include:

- a drug history
- checking for constipation/retention of urine
- asking about headache and checking the fundi
- checking for cyanosis and dehydration
- listening to the chest and checking an MSU and serum calcium.

Interventions may include antibiotics, oxygen, alteration of medication, nicotine (or alcohol) replacement, catheterization, enemas and so on. The level of investigation and intervention needs to be carefully balanced against the patients' overall condition, and their known wishes about levels of intervention. Some patients will wish to stay out of hospital at all costs; others to have every possible treatment, however invasive.

Managing confusion in palliative care: Step 3 — control the uncorrectable

Drug treatment is worth considering early, as this is such a distressing and frightening symptom for patients and their families.

Anti-psychotics are the mainstay of treatment. Haloperidol is usually suitable and has the advantage of oral tablets, capsules or suspension, and parenteral preparations suitable for subcutaneous administration (as well as intramuscular and intravenous). It is generally well tolerated, but can cause extrapyramidal syndromes. Doses range from 1.5–30 mg daily in severely disturbed and agitated patients. Typical doses are 5–20 mg daily; less in the elderly.

Benzodiazepines are a useful adjunct where there is concomitant fear or agitation.

Lorazepam 0.5–2 mg twice-daily orally or midazolam 10–100 mg per twenty-four hours via a syringe driver (start with 10 mg and titrate up according to response) reduce anxiety, although used in isolation may exacerbate confusion (see also *Chapter 3*).

Further reading

Barraclough J (1997) Depression, anxiety and confusion. *Br Med J* **315**: 1365–68

British Geriatric Society (2000) *Delirium Guidelines*. British Geriatric Society, London

Kearney M (1996) *Mortally Wounded*. Marino, Dublin

National Cancer Institute *Depression*. US National Cancer Institure review. National Cancer Institute, Bethesda, MD. Online: www.cancer.gov/cancertopics/pdq/ supportivecare/depression/HealthProfessional

National Cancer Institute *Anxiety*. US National Cancer Institure review. National Cancer Institute, Bethesda, MD. Online: www.cancer.gov/cancertopics/pdq/ supportivecare/anxiety/HealthProfessional

Stedeford (1984) *Facing Death*. Heinemann, London

Part 3
Social

14

Families

---

*No man is an island, entire of itself; every man is a piece of the
continent, a part of the main....*

    John Donne, 1624, Meditation 17, *Devotions upon Emergent Occasions*

No palliative care patient is an island; each is a piece of a family structure, a
part of a whole.

14.1 What do we mean by a family?

A family is the complex network of inter-related and interdependent people around
an individual. The relationships may be genetic, sexual and/or emotional. Modern
families defy definition. They range from huge extended structures spanning
many generations and even continents, to a single mother with one child.

A nurse was asked to sculpt a family on a training day. She chose two
parents, two children and two sets of grandparents looking on. This would be a
minority group in Britain today. Rising divorce rates and increasing birth rates
to single women have led to complex family groups. Single parent households
are common. Divorce can lead to estrangement and bitterness, not only between
ex-partners, but also between ex-family networks of uncles, aunts, cousins
and grandparents. Re-marriage by one or both partners creates new layers of
relationships to negotiate with 'ex'-family and 'step'-family, both of whom may
feel they have equal claim to the affection of and decision-making processes
around the dying person.

Bereaved family members, especially children, may find themselves caught
in divided loyalties. One woman described visiting her dying stepmother in
hospital to support her long-estranged father, while trying to protect her mother
from knowing this as she had been so hurt by what had happened years before.
The strategy worked until her mother's second husband was admitted into the
same hospital.

Stable family units may be headed by single-sex couples, widow(er)s,
grandparents, uncles and aunts.

> ### Useful strategies in complex families
>
> ❖ Draw a simple family tree (a genogram) or identify main supporters.
> ❖ Identify the next of kin.
> ❖ Identify a key person for communication. Ask the patient to assist with this; if he or she is too ill, ask the next of kin to nominate a 'family spokesperson'.

14.2 Family dynamics

Family structures are not static; they face many changes over time (see *Figure 14.2.1*).

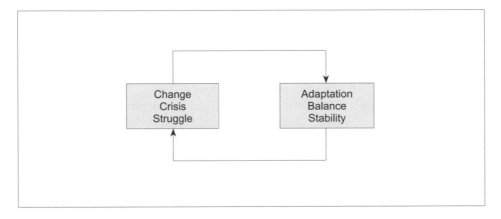

Figure 14.2.1: Family dynamics

Each change or crisis causes a shift in the balance, a loss of the familiar. A child is born, an adult finds or loses work, a major change of location occurs. Roles and support networks are altered, and through a whole variety of different coping mechanisms the family unit adapts and finds a new point of balance. Coping mechanisms may vary enormously. One family may argue and shout loudly; another may withdraw. A family may be fiercely independent and resist all offers of help despite a high level of need; another may wish maximum input for seemingly trivial need and make multiple demands on team members. We tend to judge 'normal coping behaviours' by our own standards based on our background, culture and internalized values. Families in practice, like our patients, are highly individualized and unique structures. Some families may appear utterly chaotic, yet have managed like this for many years in what for an observer seems a crisis, but is for that family a deeply familiar and stable way of life.

Useful strategies

❖ Ask how this family usually copes? Are you looking at a response to a family crisis or a longstanding behaviour pattern?

❖ Keep sight of your care goal. This is supporting this family in caring for their ill family member in the best way they can. Our words and actions should enhance that, not diminish it.

❖ If it's working, don't try to fix it.

A diagnosis of a serious illness will throw the usual family roles, relationships, assumptions and behaviours out of balance for a period until a new point of balance is found (*Figure 14.2.2*).

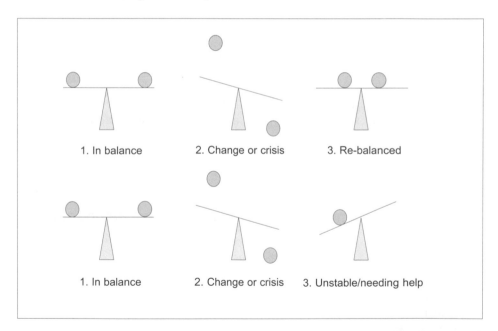

Figure 14.2.2: Impact of a serious/terminal illness on the family

⌘ Generally there is a reassessment of the whole family relationship and its meaning and value. This can bring increased appreciation and closeness; it can also sometimes produce a painful acknowledgement of gaps and deficiencies. Occasionally, this may lead to a separation.

⌘ Mutual protection is common. This can sometimes close down communication, leads to collusion and the stressful keeping of secrets. It can also sometimes lead to the premature loss of roles ('you are not well enough to do that'), and the patient's consequent sense of self-worth and meaning.

⌘ Family loyalty and a sense of duty may prevent honest disclosure and discussion of problems, such as finances.

As the patient deteriorates:

• there is a shift from coping with the impact of the disease to coping with the impending loss of the person
• familiar and long-standing roles need re-allocating. This can produce anxiety and distress, particularly if the changes are fought too long or ignored. It can be used creatively if the ill person can be encouraged to prepare and support other family members in unfamiliar tasks, such as managing the finances or preparing basic meals
• anticipatory grieving and basic self-protection may result in emotional isolation or distancing
• high levels of stress will sometimes produce increased rigidity, making problem-solving more difficult
• exhaustion is common, particularly where there is a significant care component.

It is important to stress that many families have the resources and coping mechanisms to deal with serious illness and death without needing specialist intervention or help.

14.3 Family members using different coping mechanisms

There are many different ways of coping with challenge, and many people use more than one. Common styles are:

• denial
• fighting spirit
• stoical acceptance
• hopeless resignation.

Early research suggested denial and fighting spirit were possibly associated with longer survival times, although this has not been confirmed. There is no 'right' or 'wrong' coping mechanism. A common cause of problems within a family is when there are either very different coping mechanisms, or two members of a family are at very different stages to each other in their inner journey.

> **Example**
>
> A woman was distressed at her inability to talk about her impending death with her husband and young adult daughter. Although relatively well, she was convinced she might die very soon. Her daughter could not bear to hear this and spent many of her waking hours searching the internet for possible cures.

Tension is increased in this situation by each person's belief that their way is 'right' and the other 'wrong'. Explain to the family and patient that it is common to cope differently to each other. Keep the focus on what helps the patient; 'I know it helps you a lot to keep searching for possible cures, but what your mother says she needs just now is to be able to talk a bit about what happens if a cure is not possible'. A common and useful phrase is 'prepare for the worst, but hope for the best'. This gives permission for many different coping styles. If one partner needs much more detailed information than the other, it is worth acknowledging this and negotiating agreement about how to meet the different needs; for example, 'Your husband has many detailed questions and I know you have told me you would prefer not to know any more at the moment. Would it be OK if I saw him at the surgery?'

14.4 Collusion

A family may insist a patient is not told the truth of his or her situation: 'He/she would never cope'. Rarely, the patient insists the family be not told: 'I cannot bear to see them upset — they have too much to deal with'. This leaves the team with a difficult dilemma. Sometimes the collusion is so extreme it is almost impossible to speak with the patient without an anxious family member hovering in the background.

Collusion is almost always based on:

- a genuine sense of love and protectiveness directed at the person from whom the information is being withheld (a desire to 'spare them pain')
- a self-protective urge because it is painful to watch a loved one's pain ('I can't bear to see her cry').

These are good and understandable motives. Understanding them is the key to working with collusion. We can then understand the family is not being deliberately dishonest or difficult. They are trying to help, even if the effect of their action is to increase stress and tension.

Example

John had blocked every attempt to tell his wife about her advanced ovarian carcinoma. He said it would 'finish her off' if she knew the truth, and their daughter, who lived some distance away, supported him. Elsie kept asking why her abdomen was so swollen and why she did not feel any stronger. She was increasingly agitated about this.

Tension is increased because as the suspicious partner becomes more isolated and frightened, the withholding partner interprets this as evidence of increased emotional vulnerability and inability to 'deal with the news'.

How to handle collusion

Start with the withholding partner: In the example above, collusion can be managed effectively by first acknowledging that John has his wife's best interests at heart, he knows her well and that this whole situation must be hard for him. Explain that many people in this situation exactly like him try their best to keep the diagnosis a secret to spare the other pain.

Then tell him gently that you have known Elsie for some time, and you know she is an intelligent woman. Explain your concern that some of the questions she is asking you/your team, in your experience, would make you suspect strongly that she has already guessed the truth without being told, and is maybe trying to protect him in exactly the same way. Explain this is a common reaction, particularly when a couple is close; while each means well, its effect can be to make it much harder and more frightening for both of them than 'if you were dealing with it together'.

There are then several options:

⌘ To offer to talk to Elsie and find out what she does know or guess (promising not to force information on her that she clearly does not want).
⌘ To suggest that John and Elsie talk together, offering to stay to deal with any medical questions that might arise.
⌘ To give John a little time to think things through if he is still unsure.

⌘ If you feel out of your depth, ask for help or advice from your local palliative care specialist team, who will be familiar with this sort of situation.

⌘ Rarely, it is just impossible to get open and honest communication in a family without serious, basic disruption to the family dynamics.

Remember your basic care goal. This is supporting this family to care for their ill family member in the best way they can. Our words and actions should enhance that, not diminish it. If a family have never communicated openly, it may be beyond their resource to do that now.

14.5 The distant, isolated or excluded family member

Geographical distance

⌘ Reduces communication and ability to keep up with events.
⌘ Increases anxiety.
⌘ May produce guilt — 'I should be doing more to help'.
⌘ Produces logistical problems — 'I need to book flights. When is the best time?'

All of this can produce anxious, angry or distressed telephone calls to the family doctor. As always, permission to speak to the family member must be given by the patient.

Common needs of the distant family member

⌘ Confirmation that the clinical picture is accurate and not unduly over- or under-optimistic.
⌘ Information about any further treatment plans.
⌘ Information about local support services.
⌘ 'When should I come?'. This must be the relative's decision. It is worth pointing out that regret more commonly results from arriving too late, than from arriving too early. A more meaningful visit can arise if it is not left until the patient is too ill to communicate, although this may mean staying longer, or not being present at the moment of death.

The isolated (lonely) family member

Sometimes there is only one family member. This needs to be recognized as this relative may be particularly vulnerable throughout the illness and into bereavement.

These families need additional support and may benefit from early referral to social services, support groups and other agencies.

Excluded family member: 'the outcast'

This may be secondary to a family feud or rift. It may be even more complex and be a secret lover, mistress, or covered-up homosexual relationship. These people are a vulnerable high-risk group for bereavement.

14.6 Hearing different things from different doctors (or nurses)

Different family members may see different doctors and nurses at different times. The doctors and nurses may themselves have different levels of understanding of the patient's condition and prospects. Sometimes, the information given differs significantly; it can also be heard differently. Conflicting messages increase anxiety, reduce confidence and can lead to anger, distrust and litigation.

If asked for information:

- always check what the person already knows/understands and where his or her information source was
- ensure your own facts are accurate and up to date
- communicate clearly as a team about what has been said and to whom
- try to appoint a family spokesperson.

Palliative care should be a team effort, with good communication between professionals.

14.7 The needs of the children

Children tend to be overprotected from the impact of serious illness and death. This is done in kindness, but can create problems:

* anger
* the loss of the chance to say goodbye
* feelings of exclusion and isolation
* confused feelings ('Was it my fault? Was it because I was naughty?')
* sadness.

Generally, it is best if children are given regular, simple, honest information and chance to ask questions and express feelings.

Important principles

⌘ Work through the parents. Support the parents and help the parents talk to the children, even if they choose different words and explanations to ones you would use.
⌘ Find out what the child knows.
⌘ Use simple, clear language, avoiding euphemisms.
⌘ Use play or story books.
⌘ Each child reacts differently. Children more commonly have short bursts of emotion, and may then play as though nothing is happening; this is normal.
⌘ Encourage the familiar routine and activities (this helps parents too).
⌘ Encourage the family/social network: grandparents, schoolteachers, youth leaders. They are more distant emotionally and may be good sources of stability and support.

Remember adult offspring. Research shows that adult offspring may have more anger and depression than the patient or partner.

14.8 Carers

In addition to the impact of serious illness on the family as a whole, commonly one or more family members will take on a caring role.

Who cares?

Ninety percent of the last year of life is spent at home. Three-quarters of patients will receive care from a lay carer, who may or may not share the home with them. Most of these carers are female; many of them are older. Lay carers are vital team members. One-third of patients rely on a single carer; almost half have two or three carers, such as a partner and an adult son or daughter (Ramirez *et al*, 1998). Although commonly portrayed as a burden, one-half of carers find care is rewarding, 10% find it a burden and the rest find it sometimes rewarding and sometimes burdensome.

Supporting carers

Recognition/valuing the role of carers: carers rank the GP as the person most able to make a difference to their lives. They want to be recognized as carers, be valued for their contribution and have their observations and opinions listened to.

Information needs of carers:

- 84% of carers want information on the patient's likely life expectancy
- 72% of carers want information on the extent of the illness
- 50% of carers want information on possible future complications.

Most carers express a need for regular information and updating about the patient's clinical condition, and about benefits or other support services available.

Education of carers and confidence in nursing interventions

As illness progresses, carers may take on a twenty-four-hour responsibility. They take on increasing numbers of tasks — washing, personal care, lifting, turning and transferring — which are not a usual part of everyday human relationships. Ninety percent of carers have no training in this, nor in the supervision and administration of medication. A simple introduction to and training in these tasks from district nursing staff can improve confidence and morale (see also care in the last few days of life). Supervising medication is a major source of stress for lay carers. The use of simple prescription charts, which also explain the indications for different medications and the safe use of any additional as 'required' doses, is helpful. Dosette boxes or a system of setting out the medication for the next twenty-four hours on clearly labelled saucers for patients whose fingers or eyes do not enable the use of a dosette box will assist a lay carer who is not continuously present.

Respite needs of carers

Carers cannot sustain twenty-four-hour care for long periods; they need regular, predictable time out to rest, socialize and attend to personal and domestic needs, such as their own health, the hairdressers, shopping and friendships. Potential sources of respite to explore are:

- friends/other family members
- volunteer befriending schemes
- hospice day-care services
- sitter schemes, such as the Macmillan carer scheme
- night sitting or nursing services, such as Hospice-at-Home services
- Marie Curie service
- holiday assistance
- planned inpatient respite care via a community hospital, a nursing home or a hospice.

Unreliable respite may create rather than relieve stress (leaving carers having to re-organize at short notice their own work or study routines). Carers also report ambivalence towards professional helpers. The help is valued, but it can feel hard to be 'on show' to a professional in one's own home. Well-planned and negotiated respite, introduced ideally just before it is needed, can make a big difference to the carer's ability to continue the caring role.

Emotional needs of carers

- ⌘ **Carers have higher levels of anxiety/depression than patients.**
- ⌘ Carers overestimate pain, dependency and disability of the patient.
- ⌘ 'The patient feels the pain and takes a painkiller; the carer watches helplessly and suffers'.

As well as the physical effort of caring and the need to learn a range of new skills with little support or training, the carer is usually experiencing a concomitant grief reaction.

Simply maintaining a friendly professional interest and remembering to ask about the health and welfare of the carer as well as the patient is of immense value and is remembered for many years. Recognize anxiety and depression, and treat it as vigorously as you would the patient.

Community specialist palliative care nurses have special training in supporting families and carers, from applying for benefits and grants to emotional support and counselling. Consider using their services.

Key points

❖ A family is a dynamic system, which has well-practised, unique coping mechanisms maintaining its stability.

❖ A crisis such as a serious or terminal illness stresses these coping mechanisms.

❖ Families may need to go through a period of instability as expectations and roles change before a new balance is found.

❖ Good care empowers this process, working with what works for the families rather than taking over.

❖ Caring is a paradox; both rewarding and challenging.

❖ Recognizing the contribution of carers is fundamental.

❖ Carers need information, education in the caring role, emotional support and respite.

❖ Community specialist palliative care nurses have special training in supporting families and carers. Consider using their services.

Further reading

Faulkner A, Maguire P (1994) *Talking to Cancer Patients and their Relatives.* Oxford University Press, Oxford

Ramirez A, Addington-Hall J, Richards M (1998) The carers. In: Fallon M, O'Neill B, eds. *ABC of Palliative Care.* BMJ Books, London

Sheldon F (1997) *Psychosocial Palliative Care.* Nelson Thornes, Cheltenham

Simon C (2001) Informal carers and the primary care team. *Br J Gen Practice* **51** (472): 920–3

Smith N (1990) The impact of terminal illness on the family. *Palliative Med* **4**: 127–35

15

Sexuality

For many doctors and nurses, consideration of sexuality in a palliative care setting can feel inappropriate, irrelevant, awkward and taboo. It is probably one of the least discussed areas, despite being a basic human need. Estimates of sexual dysfunction after cancer treatments range from 40–100% (National Cancer Institute, 2004). About half of women with breast or gynaecological cancer may experience long-term sexual dysfunction, as may most men after treatment for prostate cancer. Sexual problems do not tend to resolve, remaining constant and severe even a year or two after treatment, and can significantly affect quality of life. The aetiology of sexual problems is complex.

Example

Joan was Joe's main carer. He had been left paralyzed and incontinent by his spinal cord compression secondary to metastatic carcinoma of the lung. As well as preparing the meals and keeping the home clean and tidy, which she had always taken a pride in, Joan dressed and undressed Joe each day. She changed his catheter bag and washed him 'down below'. She washed him again after his struggle to evacuate his bowels when he had his enemas from the nurses. She washed him, his pyjamas, the sheets and the pretty duvet cover of their marital bed the night his bowels overflowed over everything.

Everyone admired her. The nurses saw her as a model wife and carer. One asked her in a quiet moment about how the illness had affected their relationship.

Joan's comments were: 'I just don't know who I am any more. I was his wife, his lover. Am I still a wife? I feel more like his nurse, like his mother. I'd do anything for him, but I wish I didn't have to do this. He finds it so humiliating and I can't bear him touching me anymore. That feeling has just gone.'

How often do we even ask?

All of us are sexual beings. Many of the observations to follow are about people in committed sexual relationships (whether homosexual or heterosexual). The feelings and difficulties may be even more poignant and difficult for someone who is alone, where there may also be a sense of a loss of hope for establishing a future relationship to work through.

Sexuality and sexual relationships are about much more than the act of sexual intercourse. They can include meeting needs for:

- companionship
- love
- intimacy
- sexual activity
- shared domestic arrangements
- child-rearing/parenting
- shared financial commitments.

Serious illness can impact in a number of ways. It can affect:

- physical function
- body image
- self-image
- image as a man or woman.

15.1 Physical function

General effects of illness

The fatigue, weakness and cachexia that can arise from serious illness can produce non-specific difficulty in initiating or maintaining sexual activity. Uncontrolled symptoms can compound this. Pain on movement, nausea, vomiting, halitosis, faecal incontinence, foul odours or discharges need addressing.

Specific effects of the illness

More specific problems can be anticipated and prepared for in certain situations.

Pelvic surgery and radiotherapy. For both sexes, extensive surgery for bowel cancer, gynaecological cancer or prostate cancer may lead to pelvic nerve damage and varying degrees of loss of sexual function. Loss of erectile function in men and loss of vaginal lubrication/orgasmic capability in women may result, although genital sensitivity and libido may be unaffected. Perineal scarring or partial resection of the vagina may cause dyspareunia. Radiotherapy can cause vaginal stenosis and dryness. It can cause gradual-onset erectile dysfunction after treatment for prostate cancer caused by arterial damage.

Medication effects. Some treatments may affect libido and/or erectile and orgasmic function. Hormone manipulation and 'chemical castration' for prostate cancer reduces libido and erectile function. It is not unreasonable to suppose similar effects on female sexual function with some breast cancer treatments, although there is little published literature. Spironolactone, cimetidine and tricyclic antidepressants and serotonin-specific reuptake inhibitors can sometimes cause sexual dysfunction or impotence. Opioids may also reduce libido.

15.2 Body image

Body image relates partly to the appearance of the body (how it looks to an observer), and also to how the patient sees the body, which may be coloured or distorted by how the patient feels.

General effects

Weakness, muscle wasting and cachexia will alter general appearance, as will pallor, jaundice or the yellowish discoloration of some advanced malignancies. This can be inhibiting for patient and partner, who may fear causing pain or harm. Gross Cushingoid side-effects from steroids are physically unattractive.

Specific effects

Patients with long-term urinary catheters need specific advice. Stomas, disease or surgery involving secondary sexual characteristics, such as the genitalia, perineum or breasts, and superficial discharging or fungating lesions are often difficult for patients and partners. Reconstructive surgery, prostheses and attention to well-fitting appliances can help in readjustment, although women who opt for breast conservation while rating their physical attractiveness better, do not report different levels of sexual activity or satisfaction to women opting for mastectomy. There is almost always a grief or loss reaction that patient and partner need to travel through as well. This is a sensitive area and one in which much skilful communication is needed. It can be an unrealistic expectation that a 'loving partner' can adjust quickly and easily, while also being a tower of strength for their ill lover. Support and counselling may need to be available for both.

Self-image

Much of our self-esteem and sense of meaning and belonging come from the fulfilment of the many roles each of us carries. A serious illness challenges many of the roles involved in a sexual relationship. It also challenges its duration and continuity. Either partner may avoid sexual activity as a self-protection against some of the pain of this. At the same time, the external physical changes and the altered body image can challenge how the person sees himself or herself as a sexual being. This may need revising considerably if it is based on physical appearance or a certain frequency of sexual activity.

Sexual attractiveness is valued in most societies. Sexuality is also part of the whole inner image of what it means to be a man or a woman. This is a core part of identity.

The feelings around sexual attractiveness and arousal for both patient and partner may move at a different rate. One may be anxious to reassure the other with sexual activity; they may be re-buffed because of unresolved fear and grief or it just being too soon. The huge change in roles can impact on fundamental feelings about the relationship. Caring roles can make the carer feel parental and the one cared for feel child-like. If this is not consciously recognized and addressed it may subconsciously stimulate primitive taboos against sexual contact. All these complex feelings need good communication between partners to prevent secondary anxieties and problems.

15.3 How to help

* Be willing to listen for cues to sexual or relationship problems, whatever the age of the patient.
* If patients have risk factors described above, gently enquire if the illness is interfering with their relationship in any way.

⌘ Be aware of and use local resources for body image or sexual counselling where indicated.

⌘ Optimize symptom control.

⌘ Encourage attention to personal cleanliness/grooming, alteration of clothing if body shape changes and the use of cosmetic prostheses and aids.

⌘ Encourage the ongoing expression of affection by touch and physical closeness until able to recommence sexual activity.

⌘ Encourage open communication between partners.

⌘ Explore unrealistic fears.

⌘ Exclude depressive illness.

Specific treatments

⌘ Programmed non-coital pleasuring (sometimes with encouragement of mutual self-stimulation) can assist rehabilitation if anxiety/fear are significant.

⌘ Advice on positioning if painful scar.

⌘ Specific advice for patients with ostomies (access via national organization or local stoma therapist).

⌘ Erectile dysfunction may be helped by sildenafil (Viagra®) if mild.

⌘ Severe physical dysfunction may warrant specialist referral for interventionist treatments (including prostheses).

⌘ Vaginal dryness may be helped by lubricants (eg. KY gel).

⌘ Atrophic vaginitis may respond to topical oestrogens or hormone replacement therapy.

⌘ Vaginal dilators may help after partial vaginal resection or post-radiotherapy stenosis.

⌘ Catheterized men can bend the catheter against the penis and secure it with a sheath. Other options are suprapubic catheterization and intermittent self-catheterization.

As a serious illness progresses, an increased desire for physical closeness may be accompanied by a reduced desire for sexual intercourse. The need for touch and intimacy remain. The partner can be encouraged to hold a hand, wipe a brow, to participate in the care of the patient, to hug or cuddle. Planning the care environment should recognize this need.

Key points

❖ Sexual problems are common and persistent after treatment for cancer.
❖ Suspect in patients with breast, gynaecological and prostate cancer.
❖ Aetiology is complex, and is both physical and psychological.
❖ It is important to encourage communication between partners.
❖ Unresolved sexual problems affect quality of life.

Further reading

Atkinson K (1997) Incorporating sexual health into catheter care. *Prof Nurse* **13**: 146–8

National Cancer Institute (2004) Sexuality and reproductive issues. www. cancer. gov/cancerinfo/pdq/supportivecare/sexuality (extensively referenced overview of a neglected area with direct links to citations)

Rice AM (2000) Sexuality in cancer and palliative care. *Int J Palliative Nurs* **6**: 392–7

Wells P (2002) No sex please, I'm dying. A common myth explored. *Eur J Palliative Care* **9**: 119–22

16

Legal and ethical issues

16.1 Ethical principles

Our first concern must always be the care of our patients.

Basic ethical principles are:

- first, do no harm (non-maleficence)
- second, if you can, do good (beneficence)
- respect the patient's individuality (autonomy)
- use available resources fairly and equitably (justice).

These seem admirable and simple principles. In practice, they often conflict. An individual may wish to come home to die, but the family may be exhausted and feel it is beyond their capacity to manage. Most treatments carry both the potential for harm and the potential for good. Funding issues may mean a treatment is not available for everyone who might benefit. To make a treatment available might mean other patients not having access to a particular service locally. These dilemmas become more acute where death is near.

The basic principle of respect for human life must be carefully balanced against the inevitability of death and the need for comfort and relief of suffering.

16.2 Ethical dilemmas

A dilemma is defined as:

- a situation where a choice has to be made between two equally undesirable alternatives
- a state of indecision between two alternatives

• a difficult situation, a problem (Greek — 'double premise').

In modern medicine generally and in palliative care, ethical dilemmas arise where there is no straightforward answer or decision. Treatments carry a mix of benefits and burdens. Non-treatment or non-intervention decisions also carry a mixture of benefits and burdens. A patient's concerns may differ significantly from a doctor or nurse's professional assessment of a situation. The doctor may feel further treatment is hopeless; the patient may be prepared to try anything to maximize the chance of being alive. Another patient, in the same situation, may feel that dying is a natural end to his or her life and wish as little intervention as possible, while the doctor may feel treatment is vital.

While respecting individual autonomy, futile overtreatment uses resources that would otherwise be available to others. All societies have finite resources, and a balance is needed between the good of the individual and the needs of the whole. Futile overtreatment and inadequate undertreatment of patients are undesirable. There is a need to clearly define goals of treatment in each situation and to recognize and deliver appropriate care. A balance is required between resources devoted to intervention and those available for palliation and care (*Figure 16.2.1*).

16.3 How do legal and ethical principles relate to each other?

Ethics are the moral principles we apply to our decision making. The legal framework is the framework of written rules of our society. If we transgress those rules, we may face civil or criminal prosecution (*Figure 16.3.1*).

Clinical governance may mean the practice having up-to-date copies of national and local guidelines on withholding and withdrawing life-prolonging treatment or cardiopulmonary resuscitation. It may mean team members regularly reflecting on and sharing ethical dilemmas in practice.

For difficult ethical decisions use a basic framework

⌘ Consider all the factors. Get a picture of the problem.
⌘ Start from first principles. The basic ethical principles and the relevant legal framework.
⌘ What is the overall aim or goal? Is it realistic?
⌘ Are there any alternatives?
⌘ Get other people's viewpoints.

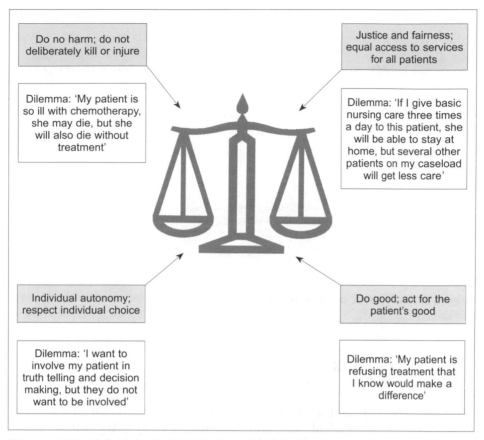

Figure 16.2.1: Principle of ethical balance in palliative care

It is important to remember that these areas are difficult because there is no clear-cut answer. Each case may throw up new factors that influence decision making in a different way. Contemporary ethics are not based on ultimate truth; ideas about right and wrong evolve and change as society changes. For example, the balance between the individual's autonomy and the needs of the whole community can differ in different cultural groups.

Ultimately, every decision we make is contained within an ethical framework as well as a rational, evidence-based practice and good professional judgment. This framework will determine what weight we give to developing our communication skills, patient choice, best or cheapest treatment in a resource-limited service, how we use our time and so on.

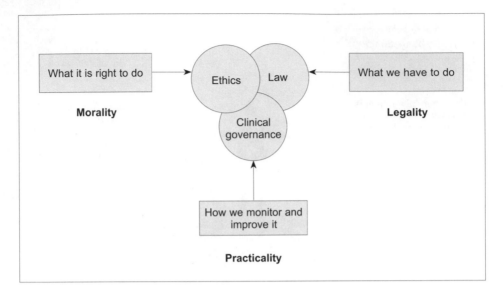

Figure 16.3.1: Ethics, legality and practicality

16.4 Truth telling

Honesty, integrity and trust are core parts of most moral frameworks. Information about a patient's condition belongs primarily to the patient, and he or she cannot be given true choice in the absence of that information. Respect for the individuality or autonomy of the patient would tell us that truth telling is important and fundamental. However, it needs to be done in an ethical way. That means:

⌘ Respecting the patient's right to information about his or her health.
⌘ Respecting the patient's autonomy on the rare occasions that he or she chooses **not** to know. A patient who says, 'I would prefer not to know that, doctor', is exercising his or her right to choice, in the same way as a patient who asks for information about every possible hazard of a treatment.
⌘ Allowing individual choice in the amount of information. Most people wish to know their diagnosis, many wish to know about treatment options, but fewer wish to know about prognosis (to which doctors and nurses frequently cannot give a certain answer), and very few indeed want detailed information about possible mechanism of death.
⌘ Being honest within ourselves about the difference between opinion ('We don't always know, but my guess would be....') and truth.

If we approach truth telling in an ethical way, we also need to make sure we are doing good, or at least doing no harm. This means:

- making sure our information is as correct as possible
- communicating in a kind and caring way
- allowing time for information to 'sink in'
- allowing the patient to adjust in the way that works best for them. One in ten people will cope best by denial. That can feel uncomfortable for the carer, who may feel it should be 'broken' to permit more open discussion. If denial is working well for the patient, we must ask whose needs we are serving by 'breaking' it
- providing a safety net — 'If you have questions/worries/concerns, the practice nurse/district nurse/palliative care nurse specialist can help you talk them through'.

16.5 Confidentiality and team working

Ethical and legal codes for doctors and nurses stress that information disclosed in a professional setting is confidential. This includes who may see the patient's record. Legally, to see the patient's notes or to hear about them at a team meeting, one must be defined as a 'health professional' for 'medical purposes'. Permission needs to be given by the patient for the information to be accessed by anyone else. There is debate about this. Policy needs to be considered in relation to reception staff, social workers, chaplaincy and so on. An ethical approach involves balancing individual autonomy and right to privacy against the fairness and justice of having access to a full range of services, which might be logistically impossible if multiple, individualized consent forms were needed for a discussion about a patient's care.

A simple question, such as 'I work as part of a team that includes... nurses, social workers, occupational therapists, physiotherapists, chaplaincy, and so on... If I think they can help, even indirectly, are you happy for me to discuss your situation with them?' can avoid much misunderstanding. Stress that all the professionals you work with are bound by professional codes of confidentiality, and make sure that is well understood in the team.

16.6 Family and friends

Giving information to family and friends without the patient's consent undermines his or her autonomy. It can also cause harm and stress important relationships.

Occasionally patients will refuse permission for relatives to be told about their condition. This raises immense problems and ethical dilemmas, particularly if the family is in a caring role:

- there is a clear distinction to make between communication necessary for the patient's care and idle gossip
- there is a clear duty to seek patient consent wherever possible or practical
- the team of professionals looking after a patient have a duty to maintain confidentiality
- the same team of professionals looking after a patient also has a duty to communicate effectively
- consent must be obtained before giving information to family or friends.
- verbal consent is adequate. A simple question such as 'Are you happy for me to answer any questions your partner and family may have about your health?' will suffice.

16.7 When patients cannot decide for themselves

Sometimes, a patient may excercise his or her autonomy by asking that the professional team make treatment decisions. Ethical decisions should then follow best practice guidelines, taking into account the individual features of the situation and any known patient preferences.

Sometimes, because of learning disability, dementia, severe communication disability or just being too ill, the patient is unable to decide. Where patients cannot decide for themselves, the duty is to try to ascertain what their wishes would have been.

First, the doctor should carefully weigh up the benefits and burdens of the intervention being contemplated. Any alternative options should also be considered.

All possible effort needs to be made to overcome communication disability. If there are doubts about mental ability, a thorough assessment is vital, including legal tests of capacity. It may be advisable to get a specialist opinion.

If the patient has a relevant advance care directive, this can give guidance. Likewise, if the patient has consistently expressed certain wishes to family or professionals, these can be taken into account. Families can be asked to try to imagine what the patient might have chosen or wanted; 'Can you imagine him as he was before all this started. What would he have said?' If the patient's wishes are still not known, the GP in charge of his or her care (or the consultant) must make the decision based on the patient's best interests.

16.8 Treatment/non-treatment decisions

There are a number of treatments that may be offered to palliative care patients that carry a complex mixture of burden and benefit. A palliative chemotherapy treatment may offer several months more life, but cause fatigue or sickness. Ureteric stenting for renal failure may extend life, but allow the underlying pelvic tumour to invade lumbar-sacral nerve roots causing an excruciating pain syndrome. A patient dying from lung cancer may be prescribed antibiotics for a chest infection, and be left with severe breathlessness at rest to endure for his last week or two of life.

⌘ Legally, any mentally competent patient has the right to refuse treatment.
⌘ Legally, there is no obligation for doctors to give a treatment that is 'futile and burdensome'.
⌘ Legally, final responsibility for which treatment is clinically indicated lies with the doctor, although the patient must consent. If consent is not possible, responsibility still lies with the doctor, who must take into account any known wishes of the patient, and also hear the family's views.

In ethical terms, we are back to the balancing of good against harm, of benefit against burden, of safety against risk. The right amount of information needs to be communicated to the patient in language they can understand, so that they are empowered to make an informed choice or can understand the reasons why a particular course of action could not be recommended. In discussing these issues with patients we need to present well-balanced information.

> Be careful with the messages given if a treatment is not appropriate. If a treatment is not possible, there is always something that can be offered to ease suffering and promote comfort. A core message is 'I shall not abandon you.

16.9 The patient who refuses treatment and advance directives

Patients may refuse treatment offered. Some patients make living wills, which are a written directive made in advance stating how they would choose to be treated in given situations, should they be unable to make a decision for themselves. Legally and ethically no patient can be treated unless they have given informed consent to the treatment. As the doctor, your duty is to ensure the patient has the information to make the decision and that he or she is of sound mind. In practice, extreme treatment refusal can cause much stress and debate for the caring team, who may feel that they are hastening death by not being more persuasive in some way. It is important to share these situations among the team, and if necessary with specialist palliative care services or colleagues from secondary care for mutual support.

Living wills are legally binding. Patients often ask their GPs to help with the wording of the wills, and for them to be filed in the GP record. The record should be distinctively tagged to alert all staff that an advance directive is in place. Legally:

- the patient should be competent when making the directive
- the patient should understand the nature and effect of the procedure the directive refers to
- the directive should be made without pressure or duress
- the patient should have anticipated the situation in which the directive is to apply.

The most common advance directives cover the course of action to be taken if the patient is incompetent with advanced dementia, head injury, malignancy or degenerative disorder, which is deemed irreversible.

Advance decisions may be made about:

- cardiopulmonary resuscitation
- treatment of intercurrent illness such as pneumonia or renal failure
- artificial nutrition or hydration
- use of strong analgesia or sedation where clinically indicated, even if this shortens life expectancy or reduces conscious level.

Even if not formally written down, this sort of discussion between patients, families and healthcare staff can facilitate best care at the end of life. It can provide immense comfort to patients to know their wishes will be honoured even when they can no longer speak.

While they must be respected, there are some real disadvantages to living wills:

- people change. It is common for patients to change their minds during the course of an illness, and a situation that they may have thought was intolerable may be completely different in the lived experience. This will become more complex where advance directives are made when the person was much younger
- not all situations can be anticipated and there may be real doubt whether the patient's condition matches his or her imagined scenario
- they cannot ever take the place of good, sensitive communication and dialogue between patient and clinical staff.

It is also important to clarify that an advance directive cannot force a doctor to offer a treatment that is futile or has no clinical indication. A patient cannot request a doctor to actively end or shorten his or her life.

16.10 Cardiopulmonary resuscitation policies

Current guidance on cardiopulmonary resuscitation (CPR) is given by the Resuscitation Council (UK), the General Medical Council (GMC) and the British Medical Association (BMA).

Key points are:

- where patients are seriously ill and death is imminent, CPR is likely to be futile and may prolong dying, cause pain and suffering and be degrading and undignified
- discussion with patients and families is acknowledged as being difficult and distressing, but CPR should be discussed 'at an early stage'
- GMC guidelines clearly state that one should usually comply with the patient's request to provide CPR, although there is no obligation to provide a treatment that you consider futile.

This leaves an ethical quagmire. There is no other situation in medicine where a doctor is asked to initiate a discussion that he or she knows may cause distress about a futile treatment that the doctor is at full liberty to withhold on the grounds of futility, but which the doctor is seemingly recommended to offer!

Not surprisingly, current policies cause confusion and concern for this group of patients. CPR is an intervention designed to provide circulatory and respiratory support for acute cardiac or respiratory arrest to allow survival so the cause of the arrest can be corrected. Death from advanced malignancy is quite different. There is progressive multi-system failure over several days and the cessation of the heartbeat and breathing are the endpoint of the natural dying process, not sudden acute events.

Palliative care patients who are otherwise well and have acute cardiac or respiratory arrest may wish for and may respond to CPR. This option should be sensitively explored, with the patient's consent, alongside some of the other difficult decisions around hydration, feeding, and so on.

Key items of information are:

- CPR refers to cardiac massage and artificial respiration, which may be followed by attempts to re-start the heart with electric shocks and/or drugs
- this usually involves emergency ambulance transfer to hospital
- family are likely to be excluded from the procedure
- for patients with acute cardiac arrest, one in four will survive resuscitation
- of these, only two-thirds will get home
- if patients opt out of this sort of intervention, they will still have access to best supportive care.

It is important to think through potential consequences of the consultation before initiating it. Are you willing to support patient choice even if it conflicts with your best professional judgment? Are you possibly giving the patient an unrealistic expectation that he or she can choose treatment 'on demand'? Is the patient likely to be too distressed by this level of information to exercise full autonomy in decision making? How will you deal with the transition from discussing CPR as an option that might be of benefit to it being futile? This is a complex balance of autonomy, beneficence, kindness, compassion and common sense.

The ethics of discussing CPR once a patient is in the dying phase of an untreatable condition is itself debatable. If the patient is clearly dying of end-stage disease, resuscitation is futile. It may be kind to gently explain this to families who may be expecting or fearful of such interventions from information in the media. It is important to be clear that decisions to avoid 'high-tech' interventions that might prolong the dying phase **do not** preclude kind and humane care that is aimed at promoting comfort and as much dignity as possible. Families may worry that they should initiate some sort of resuscitation procedure or call an emergency ambulance when death happens. It is helpful to clarify that this is not necessary for an anticipated death. Almost always this relieves anxiety.

16.11 Hydration at the end of life

A natural part of the dying process for most patients is the progressive inability to take fluids. This gives rise to questions:

- will failure to maintain hydration hasten death?
- will thirst be troublesome?
- should fluids be provided by an alternative route?
- should the nasogastric/gastrostomy fluids be continued?

As with all ethical decisions, each situation needs careful assessment by the multiprofessional team, taking full account of the views of the patient and family. The overall aim is to maximize comfort. The following information may aid decision making:

- there is no evidence to date that artificial hydration for the dying patient prolongs survival or improves comfort
- some healthcare professionals believe that reduced hydration during the dying phase may increase patient comfort by reducing bodily secretions and the need to pass urine
- a dry mouth can be eased by good mouth care more easily and less obtrusively than by artificial hydration
- if artificial hydration is considered vital, use the least invasive route. If the patient already has a nasogastric or gastrostomy tube, give small volumes down it. Otherwise, consider subcutaneous fluids
- not all dehydrated patients are dying. Consider and, where appropriate, treat correctable causes of dehydration, such as hypercalcaemia, nausea and vomiting, severe diarrhoea and over-enthusiastic diuretic therapy.

16.12 Requests for euthanasia

A request for euthanasia is one of the most difficult ethical problems and leads to much debate and polarization of opinion in both lay and professional circles. Numerous arguments have been expressed from both sides; a few examples are given in *Table 16.12.1*.

Euthanasia is sometimes divided into:

- 'active euthanasia', where an action is taken to kill the patient, such as lethal injection
- 'passive euthanasia', where treatment that would have extended life is withheld.

This is confusing. Active intervention to kill is euthanasia, and this is currently illegal in the UK. If a competent adult patient wishes treatment to be stopped, the doctor is required to comply. If the doctor feels he or she cannot comply, he or she should pass the patient into the care of another doctor. The GMC has recently published guidance on withholding and withdrawing life-prolonging treatment, which gives detailed guidance for patients who are not competent (see 'Further reading').

In practice, a request for euthanasia is a serious cry for help.

The underlying reasons need to be heard. Intractable symptoms, including the accompanying psychological and spiritual distress, need to be addressed speedily and skilfully by the multidisciplinary team and specialist resources. Sometimes it can bring much comfort for the patient to know that he or she does have some control; that while you cannot give them euthanasia they are at liberty to refuse any life-prolonging treatment, and you will do your utmost to ensure comfort and dignity to the end. If distress remains overwhelming, it is possible to offer 'time out' with short-acting sedation.

Table 16.12.1: Some arguments for and against euthanasia

Euthanasia	Arguments for	Arguments against
Autonomy	Individual choice 'Right to die' Maintains individual autonomy and integrity	Impacts on survivors/society Differs to 'right to be killed'; not a real right Reduces value of life and human ability to transcend suffering
Do no harm	Avoids intractable and unbearable suffering	Asks doctors to kill patients Possible 'slippery slope'
Do good	An easy death	Obviates development of high-quality palliative care
Fairness and justice	Happens by default now but no systematic access or regulation. Denying euthanasia disadvantages those too unwell to commit suicide, such as patients with motor neurone disease	The elderly, handicapped, vulnerable may feel under pressure to 'not be a burden'. May lose current trust in doctors and medication such as strong opioids if these are used to perform euthanasia. For the good of a minority at the expense of the majority?

16.13 Prescribing at the end of life

Sometimes, something that is done with the primary purpose and intention of doing good can carry a harmful side-effect. This is called 'double effect'. Sometimes, particularly at the end of life, acceptable levels of symptom relief may mean prescribing doses of medication that cause excessive drowsiness, sedation and may consequently shorten life.

The purpose of the medication is to relieve pain and suffering. Only good is intended, and any harmful side effect is not deliberately sought. Ideally, palliative care neither hastens nor postpones death. If harmful side effects such as excessive sedation occur, that medication should only be used after every other possible method of symptom control has been explored, and with the understanding and consent of patient and family. Ethically it can then be justified by the concept of 'double effect'. In practice this should be rare. The days of doubling doses of strong opioids to 'ease the patient's passing' are long gone and illegal.

Key points

* Almost all our decisions are influenced by ethics.
* Ethical dilemmas do not have straightforward solutions.
* Sometimes conflicting ethical principles need to be balanced.
* The overall objective is the good care of the patient, acknowledging that each situation is unique.
* Where death is inevitable, the prolongation of life must be balanced against the need for comfort and dignity in dying.
* Generally, a patient's wishes should be paramount, but no doctor is obliged to offer or carry out illegal or futile treatments.

Further reading

Cook D (1983) *The Moral Maze*. SPCK, London

Ellershaw JE, Garrard E (2000) Ethical issues in palliative care. *Medicine* **32**(4): 25–6

Finlay IJ (1994) Palliative medicine overtakes euthanasia. *Palliative Med* **8**: 271–2

General Medical Council (2002) *Withholding and Withdrawing Life-prolonging Treatments: Good Practice in Decision-making*. GMC, London

Gilbert J, Kirkham S (1999) Double effect, double bind or double speak? *Palliative Med* **13**: 365–6

Joint Working Party of the National Council for Hospice and Specialist Palliative Care Services and the Ethics Committee of the Association for Palliative Medicine of Great Britain and Ireland (1997a) Ethical decision-making in palliative care: cardiopulmonary resuscitation (CPR) for people who are terminally ill. *J Eur Assoc Palliative Care* **4**:124

Joint Working Party of the National Council for Hospice and Specialist Palliative Care Services and the Ethics Committee of the Association for Palliative Medicine of Great Britain and Ireland (1997b) Ethical decision-making in palliative care: artificial hydration for people who are terminally ill. *J Eur Assoc Palliative Care* **4**:124

Kessel AS, Meran J (1998) Advance directives in the UK: legal, ethical and practical considerations for doctors. *Br J Gen Pract* **48**: 1263–6

Randall F, Downie RS (1996) *Palliative Care Ethics: A Good Companion.* Oxford University Press, Oxford

Randall F (2001) Recent guidance on resucitation: patients' choices and doctors' duties. *Palliative Med* **15**: 449–50

Willard C (2000) Cardiopulmonary resuscitation for palliative care patients: a discussion of ethical issues. *Palliative Med* **14**: 308–12

17

A brief guide to benefits

Patients and their families experience multiple losses. The loss of income and earning capacity can be a major stress, particularly as the main carer may also have reduced working hours or given up work to be with the patient. In the bewildering upheaval of coming to terms with a life-threatening illness, patients and their families may not know who to ask for advice, or may push concerns to one side, allowing debts to mount.

Most benefits are backdated to the date the claim was received. The primary healthcare team can provide good proactive care by ensuring that all patients with a life expectancy of six months or less are given help with applying for disabled living allowance (DLA) or attendance allowance (AA) under the special rules (Form DS1500). Application packs are available from the benefits office, as are the DS1500 forms for the doctor to complete to support the application. Many practices keep a stock of these in the surgery, and the district nurse or sometimes the Macmillan nurse will often take a key role in familiarizing herself with the paperwork involved.

A range of state benefits are available, all of which can be 'topped up' with income support to provide a basic income for the household. Families on means-tested benefits or income support will almost always also qualify for help with healthcare costs. There are also grants and loans available, via the social fund for families on income support and from various charities.

After the death, help with funeral expenses is available for families receiving benefits, including housing or council tax benefit, working families tax credit, income support or income-based jobseekers allowance. Bereavement benefits are available for widows and widowers.

Brief outline of benefits

State benefits

Both patients and their carers may qualify for various state benefits. Eligibility criteria change periodically. Up-to-date advice is available from the following sources:

* Benefit Enquiry Line (for people with sickness or disability). Telephone 0800 88 22 00.
* Social worker (via the hospital offering treatment or the community social work team).
* Local welfare rights office (listed under social service and welfare organizations in the Yellow Pages or via your local authority or social services offices).
* Citizens Advice Bureau (under 'citizens' in the local telephone directory).
* Social security office (under 'benefits agency' or 'social security' in the local telephone directory.

The main benefits for the patient are listed in *Table 17.1*; the main benefit for the carer is listed in *Table 17.2*.

All patients with a life expectancy of six months or less will qualify for DLA (if <65 years of age) or AA (if >65 years of age), under the special rules. There is no three-month or six-month qualifying period to serve for this group of patients. No formal medical examination is needed, and application can be made by the carer on behalf of the patient. Claims under the special rules are prioritized and will often be processed in ten to fourteen days.

People on low income may also qualify for means-tested benefits, and carers <65 years may be able to claim the carers' allowance. If in doubt it is well worth claiming.

Help with healthcare costs

Means-tested assistance may be available to help with prescription charges, travel to hospital, wigs and fabric supports. Leaflets HC81 (SG) *Free Prescriptions* and HC11 *Help with Healthcare Costs* give guidance.

Table 17.1. State benefits for the patient

Non-means tested

Disabled living allowance (DLA) or Attendance allowance (AA)	DLA <65 years AA >65 years	Fast track to the higher rate of both benefits if claimed under the special rules. Use the usual claim pack; doctor needs to complete form DS1500 to confirm terminal illness *Not means tested or taxable.* Gives additional premiums to income support, housing and council tax benefits

Means tested

Incapacity benefit (IB) or	For those with sufficient national insurance contributions	Long-term rate paid after 28 weeks for terminally ill (instead of 52 weeks)
Income support (IS)	For those who cannot claim IB and/or to 'top-up' other benefits	DLA, AA or IB awards give a 'disability premium', which may make someone eligible for income support who previously was not People on income support become eligible to apply for loans or grants from the social fund
Housing benefit Council tax benefit	For those on income support or low income	Income-related

Table 17.2. Main benefit for the carer

Carers' allowance	For carers aged 16 or over	Person cared for must be receiving middle/higher rate of DLA or AA Care must be needed ≥35 hours per week Carer can earn up to £79 per week (April, 2004) Allows a 'carer's premium' on other benefits, national insurance premiums to be paid and spares carer from 'signing on'

Going into hospital affects benefits

Disability living allowance and attendance allowance **stop** after four weeks in hospital; they restart on discharge. The recipient must inform the DSS in Blackpool to avoid overpayment.

Income support, incapacity benefit and retirement pension are reduced after six weeks. The recipient must notify the benefits agency to avoid overpayment. Mobility allowance remains if there is a contract with Motability.

Overpayments have to be paid back. This can cause unwanted problems with debt, and is better avoided.

Grants

⌘ The social fund makes grants for additional expenses, such as bedding or household items, which cannot be resourced from existing benefits.

⌘ To make a claim, the claimant must be on income support or jobseekers allowance. It can also sometimes provide loans. Application forms are available from the benefits agency.

⌘ Macmillan Cancer Relief makes grants for people with cancer facing financial hardship. Application is usually made by the Macmillan nurse or social worker, who can give further information.

⌘ CLIC/Sargent Cancer Care makes grants for children with cancer.

⌘ The Independent Living Fund can help with the costs of care at home. Application is made through social services.

Overview of benefits after the patient's death

Funeral expenses

Funeral expenses payment can be made to families receiving qualifying benefits, which include housing or council tax benefit, working families' tax credit, income support or income-based jobseekers allowance. Claims must be made within three months of the death on a form available from the benefits agency.

Bereavement benefits

Bereavement benefits are available to widows or widowers whose spouse paid national insurance contributions:

- a lump sum is payable on the death
- a widowed parents' allowance is available for families with dependent children who would qualify for child benefit
- a bereavement allowance is payable for the first fifty-two weeks after the death for widows or widowers aged forty-five years or over.

Key points

❖ Financial problems for cancer patients are common.

❖ All patients with a life expectancy of six months or less will qualify for disabled living allowance or attendance allowance under the special rules (form DS1500), and this will add a premium to any other benefits they receive.

❖ Other benefits and help with healthcare costs are available to patients on low incomes.

❖ Carers over sixteen years of age may qualify for carers' allowance.

❖ If in doubt, apply.

❖ Advise patients and families to inform the DSS (Blackpool) and the benefits agency if admitted to hospital.

18

Palliative care for minority groups

A recurring theme in this book has been the uniqueness of each life and each death, which in practical terms requires sensitive and individualized care. Within this, while wishing to avoid over-generalization, some minority groups have significantly different needs.

18.1 Stereotypes

While it is helpful to be aware that these different needs may exist, we also need to be aware of the dangers of assuming and stereotyping. Stereotypes are collections of beliefs and associated value judgments we all carry about groups of individuals. This may be on the basis of age, occupation, gender, marital status, social class, race, religion, physical or mental ability and so on. Stereotypes lead to false assumptions. Despite this, many 'educated professional people' (another stereotype) may observe themselves speaking in baby language to someone who is old and hard of hearing; assuming a professional colleague is magically 'better able to cope' with their impending death and its attendant grief and loss than someone without medical knowledge; or that a patient with an Asian name will automatically follow certain customs.

Specialist palliative care services in the UK are not well used by ethnic minority groups. Service development for children is patchy. There is evidence that while almost two-thirds of cancer deaths occur in social class 4 and 5, these lower social groups are proportionally less likely to use inpatient hospice facilities. Most hospice deaths are from the middle classes. There is no systematic provision for prisoners or people with learning disability, although there are encouraging pilot projects, led with vision.

Primary care teams have a key role in coordinating care for these minority groups.

18.2 Children

The general principles of adult palliative care apply, but children's palliative care differs from adults in a number of significant ways:

⌘ Far fewer children die or have life-threatening illness than adults. This means few GPs, district nurses or adult specialist palliative care teams will have experience with children's palliative care.

⌘ Children's cancers have cure rates of around two-thirds, which is much higher than for adults. Treatments are much more likely to be centralized in tertiary referral centres that may be at some distance.

⌘ Primary care teams have much less involvement than with adults. A decision that the child is dying is usually made much later in the illness, when child, family and staff of the tertiary centre have formed strong bonds. Often this is where the child dies. If they die at home, the primary care team may need to build trust and relationships rapidly, and a strong link with the tertiary centre is vital.

⌘ Most palliative care for children is for chronic, life-limiting illness. This carries some of the challenges of unpredictability and uncertainty that have been described for adult non-cancer palliative care. There are further challenges if the child survives to outgrow paediatric services, in making the transition into appropriate adult services.

⌘ Children's life-limiting illnesses are degenerative disorders such as metabolic disorders, neurodegenerative disorders, muscular dystrophies and cystic fibrosis or chronic organ failure from cardiac pathology, renal failure or hepatic failure. Children also die from severe multiple disability. This means that the child is likely to have a rare, complex illness that the family comes to know much more about than the primary healthcare team. This can lead to frustration and loss of confidence for both. Good liaison with specialist nursing teams where available and specialist centres is vital.

⌘ The time course of these illnesses can extend over many years, and the impact on families is enormous. Respite facilities are patchy, and the small network of 'children's hospices' that exist may be a considerable distance geographically. Medical support for them is often from a local general practice.

⌘ Many paediatric services have or are developing outreach specialist nursing services that can support GPs and district nurses as well as children and families. Diana nursing teams are in place in a number of parts of the UK serving a similar function, although they may be freestanding, linking with several paediatric units and serving a defined geographical area.

⌘ Paediatric palliative care is developing as a specialty, and models of service provision/are being actively considered in many parts of the UK.

⌘ Primary care providers are an important part of the debate.

18.3 Temporary residents

Temporary residents fall into two main groups:

- patients who are visiting family or on holiday in the area who need medical or nursing attention
- patients who have come to the parental home or a child's home to die. This can happen in a variety of circumstances, but is a relatively common occurrence for younger people dying of acquired immunodeficiency syndrome (AIDS), where the partner has already died.

The challenges are similar for both groups. There is often urgent need to access accurate diagnostic and up-to-date medical information from the usual doctor and/or hospital. There is the need to build relationship and trust. Records can be fast-tracked, and often both the usual GP and the hospital will send photocopies of key communications.

18.4 Immigrants

The needs of first-generation immigrants are often different to the needs of well-established ethnic minority groups. Depending how long the immigrant has been in the UK, areas of concern can be as follows.

Communication

There may be language difficulties and the need for interpreters. The use of family interpreters, particularly the use of children, is fraught with problems. In reality it is often unavoidable, but there needs to be a good awareness of its limitations, particularly where items of an intimate or emotional nature are concerned. Where interpreters are used, this can also cause challenges for small communities.

> An interpreter was needed for a private Cantonese-speaking lady who was depressed with multiple health and social problems. The only Cantonese-speaking interpreter the local hospital had listed was a close friend of her husband.

If the interpreter is not also regularly involved in health care, he or she may need some help and preparation. If parts of the consultation are distressing, the interpreter may need some support and de-briefing afterwards.

Social situation

Presence or absence of key family members, housing and economic stability are important factors. Sometimes key family members are on another continent. There may be reliance on the patient's income by relatives overseas.

Degree of integration/assimilation

This may range from still being part-way through a major adjustment reaction after a period of trauma (it is rare for immigration to occur without reason), to feeling 'at home' in the UK. Even for well-established immigrants, the prospect of serious illness/death can set up feelings of dislocation and a yearning for what is felt to be home.

Different illness behaviours

We all experience ethnocentricity and the belief that our own model of illness and help-seeking behaviour is the most appropriate. Behaviours during illness draw heavily on learned experience from parents and peers in early life. Being brought up in a culture that somatizes emotional distress or stresses the good of the whole family above the individual need is not necessarily better or worse than some of our own cultural eccentricities. Problems arise when these behaviours are misinterpreted by UK 'norms'. If you are working in an area with immigrant communities, learn about the commoner illness behaviours and what they mean.

Gender issues

Be as sensitive as is realistically possible to gender issues. Some cultures prefer same-sex healthcare workers or chaperones; all cultures are sensitive to intimate examinations, which should be carefully explained, properly consented, performed gently and adequately chaperoned.

Use of traditional medicines

Many cultures have traditional systems of medicine, which first-generation immigrants may place a lot of faith in (as may growing numbers of the native UK population). Ask about traditional healers and ask the patient to show you everything they are taking, including herbs and medicines that are not from the hospital. Generally, traditional medicines can complement Western scientific medicine. There is, however, potential for drug interactions, particularly with herbal remedies. Many patients will agree to stop a herbal treatment temporarily, for example while undergoing chemotherapy if they understand the reasoning.

Religious customs

Most societies are pluralistic, and more than one religion is practised in most countries of the world. Do not assume that religion and ethnic origin are the same. Many Arabs are Christian, some white British people are Buddhist, Hindu or Muslim. There are customs that originate from where individuals grew up, and customs that are part of religious practice. Historically, religions have tended to spread by 'grafting' themselves onto the pre-existing cultural practice. Thus, the 'same' religion in different countries will have differences in tradition and practice. This can be seen close to home in the different ways and dates Christmas is celebrated in Europe; if in doubt, ask.

Well-established ethnic groups

A culture is 'the distinctive customs, achievements, products, outlook, etc, of a society; the way of life of a society or group'. Culture can be completely independent of race or ethnic origin. Ethnicity on the other hand refers to 'sharing a distinctive cultural and historical tradition, often associated with race, nationality or religion by which the group identifies itself and others recognize it. This often, but not always, includes shared racial characteristics'.

Generally, as immigrant ethnic groups assimilate into the host society over several generations, there is an acquisition of some or all of the cultural characteristics of the host society. There is good evidence at present that black and ethnic minority groups in Britain do not use specialist palliative care services to the amount that could be anticipated from population numbers. It also appears that problems commonly arise around:

- communication
- religious and spiritual issues
- gender issues
- suitability/location of facilities
- availability of healthcare workers of different ethnic origins.

Most palliative care information and practice has been derived from work with white British people. Even in simple areas, such as breaking bad news, communication and information giving, there is evidence of differences in need and preferred practice.

Established ethnic minority groups will have community networks, leaders and representatives who can help inform culturally-sensitive practice.

18.5 People who are sensory impaired

Those who are blind, partially sighted or deaf have special needs. National associations for the blind and the deaf have local branches that can provide support services, translating written information onto tape or providing interpreters proficient in sign language. The comments made above about interpreters apply equally to the sensory impaired, who should not need to rely on family for all their communication needs. There needs to be particular care with medication identification for the visually impaired. Social service departments can be good resources, as can ophthalmology and ear, nose and throat departments, voluntary organizations and the local sensory-impaired community.

18.6 People with learning disabilities

Specific issues arise around communication and competence in decision making. The spectrum of learning disabilities varies. It is important to establish the patient's competence to understand information and to be involved in decision making. This will usually involve the multiprofessional team and may need specialist input. As in general palliative care, key family members need to be involved, engaged and informed. Information needs to be given appropriately to the patient's understanding and ability.

Emotional responses, worry, depression and fear can emerge. They may present in atypical ways, such as regression, soiling, repetitive behaviour, self-mutilation, picking, self-induced vomiting. Have a high index of suspicion. A good question is 'If this person could communicate normally at this moment, what do I think they would say from what I know of their medical problems and what I am told by those caring for them about any alterations in their usual behaviour?' The same applies to physical symptoms. If you know the patient has carcinoma of the breast that has metastasized to bone, ask for features that might indicate pain. Is the patient as mobile as usual? Are they sleeping normally? Are they agitated or grimacing? Medicate in the same way you would for a patient who can communicate clearly and observe the response.

18.7 Travellers ('gypsies')

Palliative care for this community is challenging. These patients often have:

- no regular medical attendant
- incomplete and patchy medical records
- patterns of non-attendance for clinics or other interventions
- high rates of smoking, alcohol or substance abuse
- no fixed address for service delivery (half live in caravans, half move in and out of housing), complicated by evictions from illegal sites
- poor living environments and low socioeconomic position
- discrimination, marginalization and harassment
- higher morbidity and mortality than other ethnic minority groups (yet not measured in most routine health service/census data).

Postcode-based services and developments are unlikely to address travellers' needs. Presentation may be to NHS walk-in centres, as temporary residents at nearby GP surgeries or to accident and emergency departments.

Information for travellers on accessing health services is available from http://www.gypsy-traveller.org/health/access.htm, including contact details for all NHS walk-in centres.

Care may need to be *ad-hoc* and proactive, working with traditional Romanic gypsy beliefs and behaviours, which tend to stress the importance of the family, the Romani community and independence, and to vigorously avoid bureaucracy and authority. There is a strong case for being as thorough as possible in a single consultation, in the knowledge that a return visit is unlikely. A basic patient-held record and, if permission is given, identifying and telephoning through to the next health worker may produce better continuity.

18.8 Prisoners

Traditionally, prisoners have not featured in palliative care programmes, possibly because the numbers dying in prison have been small. That is changing with high rates of drug abuse and AIDS. Prisoners are isolated from society. Family support may be minimal. Psychiatric disturbance is much more common than in the general population. British prisons are just starting to follow a lead from the USA in developing programmes allowing adequate levels of symptom control, emotional and spiritual support and volunteer visiting programmes for prisoners who are dying.

Key points

- While avoiding assumptions and stereotyping, it must be recognized that some minority groups have specific needs.
- Children's palliative care deals with a different spectrum of illness to that of adults, and is still developing as a specialty.
- Children are more likely to have a rare, complex illness, needing care over a longer period of time, and which the family may come to know more thoroughly than the primary care team.
- Good liaison is vital.
- Professional interpreters may be needed for the sensory impaired, or for those with insufficient skill in spoken English to express themselves.
- Family interpreters have limitations when subjects of an intimate or emotional nature are being discussed.
- Be aware of common illness behaviours, gender issues, use of traditional medicines and culturally sensitive practice.
- If learning disability precludes verbal communication, intelligently interpret what is known about the illness and observable changes in the patient's behaviour to plan treatment.

Further reading

Community Practitioners and Health Visitors Association (2001) *Tackling Health Inequalities*. Community Practitioners and Health Visitors Association, London

Doyal L, Cameron A, Cemlyn S, Nandy S (2002) *The Health of Travellers in the South-West Region: a Review of Data Sources and a Strategy for Change*. School for Policy Studies, University of Bristol and Mary Shaw, South West Public Health Observatory, Bristol

Firth S (2001) *Wider Horizons: Care of the Dying in a Multicultural Society*. National Council for Hospice and Specialist Palliative Care Services, London

Goldman A (1998) ABC of palliative care: special problems of children. *Br Med J* **316**: 49–52

Grace Project (2004) Palliative care in prisons. www.graceprojects.org

Parkes CM, Laugani P, Young B (1997) *Death and Bereavement across Cultures*. Routledge, London and New York

Part 4
Spiritual care

19

Holistic care and the cancer journey

19.1 The patient as a whole person

In practice, this means that as well as the physical aspects of the disease process, the patient will experience change in the mental and spiritual domains. The mental domain includes conscious thought processes (information, reasoning, problem solving) and emotional responses (feelings about events). The spiritual domain is where the different aspects of the experience are drawn together and integrated into something that has meaning for the individual (*Figure 19.1.*).

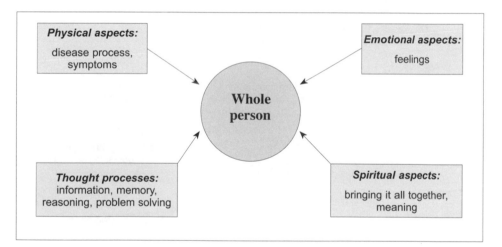

Figure 19.1: In palliative care the 'whole person' should be considered

19.2 The experience of serious illness as a journey

Cancer has been described as a journey, and the concept is applicable to any serious illness or event. The journey is travelled on several levels, corresponding to the four domains in *Figure 19.1*.

The 'biomedical journey' is worth mapping when the aim is to improve organizational aspects of patient care, for example referral times. It may also aid identification of points of maximum vulnerability.

The 'biomedical journey' (Figure 19.2.1)

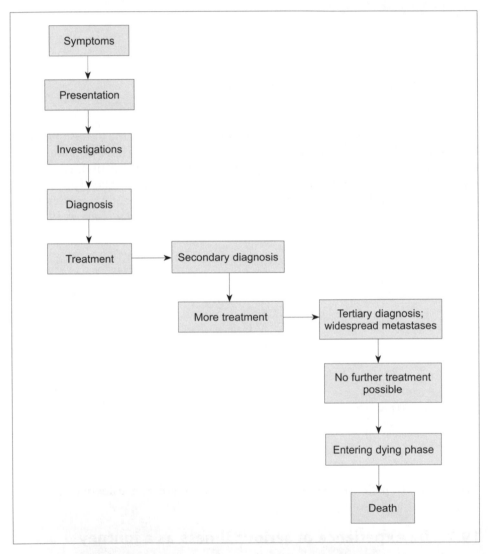

Figure 19.2.1: The physical (biomedical) cancer journey

- ⌘ The first stage of the journey is from symptoms to diagnosis.
- ⌘ The second stage travels from diagnosis through treatment, and for cancer patients to end of treatment and thereafter.

⌘ For cancer patients, there may be further stages of secondary diagnosis/ tertiary diagnosis and end-of-treatment decisions.

⌘ The final stage of the journey for the patient is the dying phase and death, but for the family there is another stage — bereavement.

At the same time as the physical (biomedical) journey, the patient is also experiencing an often profound inner journey.

The inner journey (Figure 19.2)

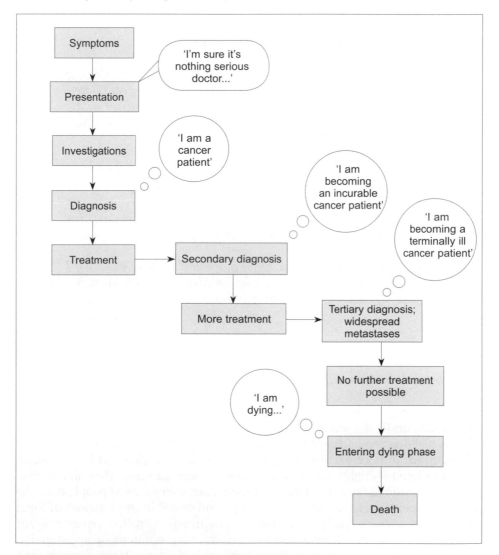

Figure 19.2.2: The inner journey: points of transition

The inner journey is the series of transitions or identity shifts patients need to make as they radically alter their view of themselves and their future.

Health professionals need to understand this journey and attention needs to be given to the inner journey and the levels on which it is operating:

- **thought processes** — giving appropriate information, facilitating patient-centred problem-solving skills
- **emotional** — anticipating and facilitating emotional expression (eg. 'how are you feeling about this?')
- **spiritual** — empathic listening; creating safe space; signposting to sources of support.

These identity shifts can be traumatic and overwhelming.

It's very silly but cancer becomes everything. If you can't sleep, get a sore elbow, develop a rash shaving, somehow it all gets related to cancer. Cancer takes over your life. You have to resist it with your whole being, your past, present and future. When everything becomes cancer you lose track of yourself.

For a while I didn't know what was pathology, pharmacology, psychology, astrology or any other 'ology'. It was all just cancer. I let cancer dictate and make all the rules. Cancer eats up your sanity. Cancer eats up your diligence. It made me dependent. The realization of that, though, was very powerful.

I'm sure I could have slipped into a perpetual cycle of cancer if I hadn't woken up to the fact that it had robbed me of my identity. The awareness of that was a regaining of power.

Patient with cancer

The journey is dynamic

An identity shift, in common with all transition, involves loss, the grieving of that loss, the acceptance of the loss and the integration of the new. This cycle is described in more detail in *Chapter 23: Grief, mourning and bereavement*. The associated thoughts, feelings and emotions are not static; they do not arise in a neatly ordered fashion. They are complex and dynamic and people describe shifts between anger, despair, sadness, hope and denial in short periods of time. A common analogy that people easily recognize is a 'roller-coaster ride' of external events with different items of information, opinions or investigation results pushing them from hope to despair and back again. If this is taken with the inner emotional roller-coaster of feelings, it becomes easier to understand why most patient groups see the wider communication and support issues around cancer and other life-limiting illness as being of vital importance to their ability to get through difficult physical treatments.

19.3 Holistic care

Holistic care endeavours to respond to physical, mental and spiritual need in an individualized, patient-led way that is appropriate for where that patient is on his or her journey. Holistic care is different to just offering access to a complementary therapist or counsellor, although the popularity of these interventions may well relate to their ability to respond to non-physical domains of need. It is the ability to see and respond to the whole human being in front of us and side-by-side, engage in a dialogue.

Some patients may need a whole range of complementary therapies, some may meet all their care needs within the family network, and others might choose to talk to you from time to time, not seeking a prescription or a careful pain assessment, but just wanting to be heard.

Key points

❖ The patient is a whole person.
❖ The experience of serious illness is a journey.
❖ The journey is dynamic.
❖ Holistic care endeavours to respond to physical, mental and spiritual need in an individualized, patient-led way that is appropriate for where that patient is on his or her journey.

20

Complementary therapies

Complementary medicine is the broad domain of healing resources that encompasses all health systems, modalities and practices and their accompanying theories and beliefs, other than those intrinsic to the politically dominant health system of a particular society or culture in a given historical period.

Cochrane Collaboration

There is a bewildering range of complementary therapies. There is good evidence that they are popular with patients, that their popularity is growing, that they are used by cancer patients (particularly younger patients of higher social class) and that patients value the holistic approach and therapeutic relationship, which gives them a greater sense of control.

Not all doctors or nurses can be familiar with all therapies, yet they may be asked to advise on or refer for this sort of intervention. Where training is available it may be patchy or superficial. There are no clear guidelines for training and competency requirements for qualified health professionals who may wish to use a complementary therapy in their work. Many patients may use these therapies without letting their family doctor know. There is a lack of research into interactions between therapies and conventional treatments. Almost certainly, better communication with, respect for and familiarization with different treatment approaches will lead to an enhanced partnership between orthodox and complementary health care, to the advantage of both groups of practitioners who have much to learn from each other. Of greater importance is the advantage to patients, who are going through experiences that deeply impact on every level of their being, of having access to expert multidisciplinary care.

20.1 Ways of classifying complementary therapies

Classification of complementary therapies according to organization, regulation and research base

The 1999–2000 British House of Lords select committees report on complementary and alternative medicine divided therapies into three groups (*Table 20.1.1*).

The select committee report also refers to group 3b 'other alternative disciplines', which includes therapies such as crystal therapy, dowsing, kinesiology and radionics. These will not be discussed further.

Table 20.1.1: Classification of complementary therapies into three groups

	Characteristics	Examples
Group 1		
Alternative therapies	• Professionally organized/regulated	• Acupuncture
	• Some evidence base	• Chiropractic
	• May be available within NHS	• Homeopathy
		• Herbal medicine
Group 2		
Complementary	• Not yet regulated	• Aromatherapy
therapies	• Not well researched	• Massage
	• May be available within NHS	• Hypnotherapy
		• Counselling
		• Reflexology
		• Healing
Group 3a		
Other alternative disciplines	• Traditional healthcare systems	• Ayurdevic medicine
		• Traditional Chinese medicine
		• Chinese herbal medicine

This classification allows the doctor or nurse to assess where a therapy sits in relation to the current orthodox UK model for ensuring regulated practice. It is not so helpful in providing a practical framework for which therapy might help in different situations, and whether a therapy might need more careful monitoring in an individual situation.

Classification of complementary therapies based on type of therapy

Basically, this divides complementary therapies into those where pharmacologically active products are taken into the body, those where pharmacologically harmless substances are ingested, touch therapies, talking therapies and creative therapies (*Table 20.1.2*). This allows a broad assessment of any potential for harm from the therapy itself and from interactions with other treatments, and can start to give broad guidance on which therapy might help when.

Classification of complementary therapies based on patient's current energy level

Dr Rosy Daniel describes a practical model for selecting complementary therapies based on where the patient is in his or her overall energy or vitality (based on work at the Bristol Cancer Help Centre over a number of years) (*Figure 20.1.1*).

As the energy level drops in response to the illness, the physical treatments, the shock of the diagnosis and the subsequent loss of expectations and major identity shift, it can fall below a critical level (about 30%). When energy is as low as this, Dr Daniels suggests that not only is the body more vulnerable to intercurrent infection and easily fatigued, but there is also a fatigue of the spirit. The patient may become depressed and feel they have no control over things. They may become fearful and anxious, sleep poorly and resort to unhealthy methods of combating stress, such as alcohol, tobacco, and food or drug abuse. Sometimes this can coincide with recovery from surgery or the end of chemotherapy; as the adrenaline that kept the patient fighting on diminishes, the true depth of exhaustion is felt. This often also coincides with a withdrawal of medical support as clinic visits become less frequent, adding to the sense of isolation. At such low energy levels, self-help is almost impossible until the patient's vitality restores either slowly with the passage of time or can be restored by therapies, which enhance energy and well being. This receiving phase is necessary for patients to recover to a point where they can start to help themselves (*Figure 20.1.2*).

When energy is low, therapies are chosen that are more passive on the part of the recipient, who is as keen to 'let go' and allow the deep relaxation and restoration of the chosen therapy to have its effect. Using this model, therapies can be selected on the basis of the patient's current energy level (*Table 20.1.3*).

Table 20.1.2: Classification of complementary therapies based on type of therapy

Type of therapy	Examples	Potential harm?	Minimize harm by:
Pharmacologically active substance ingested	Herbalism Chinese herbal medicine	Potential for drug interactions: database incomplete. Side-effects possible	Discuss in detail with prescriber
	Vitamin hyper-supplementation	Most commonly vitamin C overdose: gastrointestinal disturbances	Encourage sensible dosage regimen
Pharmacologically harmless substance ingested	Homeopathy Flower essences	Generally harmless[*]	Encourage use of homeopathy as a complementary treatment rather than as an alternative
Touch therapies	Massage Reflexology	Rare, provided well-trained therapist following protocol	Exclude bleeding tendency/ thrombocytopenia Exclude patients with thrombosis/sepsis /extensive or painful skin lesions/pyrexia
	Aromatherapy	Potential systemic and skin reactions to essential oils	Use professionally trained therapists who are members of the appropriate professional body[**]
	Healing	No harmful effects	
	Reiki	No harmful effects	
	Therapeutic touch	No harmful effects	
Talking therapies	Counselling	Generally safe	Use professionally trained therapists who are members of the appropriate professional body[**]
	Affirmations	Generally safe	
	Hypnotherapy	Generally safe	
	Visualization	Generally safe	
Creative therapies	Music therapy	Generally safe	
	Art therapy	Generally safe	
	Writing therapies	Generally safe	

[*]Homeopathy may temporarily exacerbate the symptom it is prescribed for. This is called proving, and is said to indicate effectiveness of remedy
[**] Information available from the Foundation for Integrated Medicine www.fimed.org or the National Association of Primary Care www.primarycare.co.uk

20.2 Popular complementary therapies for palliative care patients

The commonest therapies used by patients with cancer are healing therapies (Reiki, therapeutic touch, healing), relaxation/visualization and dietary modification. The commonest therapies offered by palliative care services are massage and aromatherapy. Acupuncture and hypnotherapy are sometimes used for symptom relief.

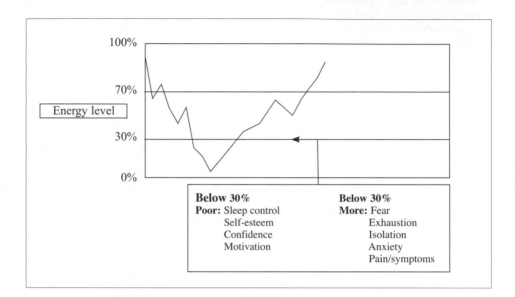

Figure 20.1.1: Dr Daniel energy graph. Reproduced with permission of Dr Daniel

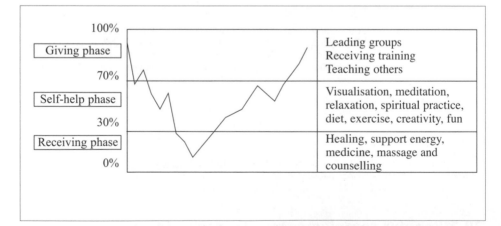

Figure 20.1.2: The Dr Daniel energy graph. Reproduced with permission of Dr Daniel

Table 20.1.3: Selection of complementary therapies based on the patient's energy level

Is your current energy:	A helpful therapy might be:	This involves:
<30%	Healing	No touch or light touch. Often a feeling of
	Reiki	warmth, tingling and deep relaxation
	Therapeutic touch	Client remains fully clothed
	Homeopathy	Taking tablets (remedies)
	Shiatsu	Touch/pressure/movement of body and limbs while fully clothed
	Reflexology	Pressure/massage of soles of the feet
	Massage	Areas being massaged are uncovered (client will undress for full massage, but be covered with towels)
	Aromatherapy	Aromatherapy massage includes the use of scented oils
	Supportive counselling	Talking one-to-one with a skilled counsellor
30–70%	Relaxation	Learning to deeply relax the body
	Visualization	Using the imagination to picture a positive goal
	Meditation	Learning to still the mind on a regular basis
	Creative therapies	Music, drama, art, writing, journal-keeping, gardening
>70%	Any	

Referral and access

Most patients with cancer using complementary therapies would prefer the referral to come from a doctor. A substantial number of GP practices provide some complementary therapies, either by interested doctors or nurses or by employing therapists for in-house sessions. Issues to consider are as follows.

Referral to complementary therapists who are also registered doctors or nurses:

✖ Therapist is fully accountable to relevant statutory regulatory body (eg. General Medical Council/Royal College of Nursing).
✖ Check the practitioner has appropriate training in therapy (not just a short introductory course).
✖ Ideally, the therapist should be a member of the appropriate complementary therapy organization.

Referrals to other complementary therapists:

⌘ Check suitably qualified/competent in therapy offered
⌘ GP retains responsibility for managing patient's care
⌘ Access to necessary conventional treatment must be maintained
⌘ If patient refuses conventional treatment, this must be recorded in the
   medical notes.

**Key issues for non-medically qualified complementary therapists
employed by a GP practice:**

❖ Qualification, registration, insurance.

❖ Consent to treatment; refusal to treat.

❖ Medical responsibility.

❖ Documentation.

❖ Education and training.

❖ Quality standards, audit, research.

❖ Health and safety, infection control.

Recommendation of complementary therapists without formal referral:

⌘ GP should be satisfied that the therapist is competent in the therapy
   offered.

Overall, there is little evidence of harm from complementary therapies, provided they are used alongside conventional therapy, rather than replacing it. There have been no claims or cases sustained against doctors who have delegated aspects of care to complementary therapists (2000). Their role appears strongest in those aspects of supportive care where doctors and nurses can sometimes feel powerless. For the right patients, complementary therapies can be a helpful adjunct.

Other questions the primary healthcare team may face

There are hundreds of complementary and alternative products available in the UK aimed at patients with cancer, including homeopathic and herbal formulations. Patients may query these with the healthcare worker. They can vary from shark's cartilage to mistletoe extract. The US National Cancer Institute (www.cancer.gov) has a good and up-to-date website (www.cancer.gov/cancer_information/list.aspx?), which provides detailed information on the current knowledge and evidence base for some of these products, including reference lists, and is a recommended resource.

Key points

❖ Complementary therapies are popular with patients, who value the sense of personal control and the therapist-patient relationship.
❖ Therapies can be classified according to the level of evidence/regulation, the type of therapy/safety and the patient's level of energy.
❖ The more popular therapies are not ones with the greatest evidence base or regulation.
❖ There is little evidence of harm from most therapies.
❖ Improved communication between complementary and conventional practitioners would enhance patient care.
❖ Where therapies are used, practitioners need to be adequately trained, competent and operate to professional standards.

Further reading

Barraclough J (2001) *Integrated Cancer Care*. Oxford University Press, Oxford
Bristol Cancer Help Centre (1999) *Meeting the Needs of People with Cancer for Support and Self-management*. Report on Focus Group Study. Bristol Oncology Centre/Department of Sociology, University of Warwick/Bristol Cancer Help Centre
Daniels R (2001) Holistic approaches to cancer: the general principles and the assessment of the patient. In: Barraclough J, ed. *Integrated Cancer Care*. Oxford University Press, Oxford
Daniels R (2003) *Bristol Cancer Centre: Living with cancer and feeling good*. Constable and Robinson, London

Department of Health (2000) *Complementary Medicine: an Information Pack for Primary Care Groups*. Download from www. fimed.org or www. primarycare. co.uk

Downer SM, Cody MM, McCluskey P, Wilson PP, Arnott SJ, Lister TA, Slevin (1994) Pursuit and practice of complementary therapies by cancer patients receiving conventional treatment. *Br Med J* **309**: 86–9

House of Lords (2000) *Science and Technology — sixth report. Complementary and Alternative Medicine*. The United Kingdom Parliament, London

Owen DK, Lewith G Stephens CR (2001) Can doctors respond to patients' increasing interest in complementary and alternative medicine? *Br Med J* **322**: 154–7

Featherstone C, Forsyth L (1997) *Medical Marriage: The new partnership between orthodox and complementary medicine*. Findhorn Press, UK

Rees L (2001) Integrated medicine. *Br Med J* **322**: 119–20

Vincent C, Furnham A (1994) Complementary medicine: state of the evidence. *J Roy Soc Med* **92**: 170–7

Zollman C, Vickers A (1999) What is complementary medicine? *Br Med J* **319**: 693–6

21

Religious needs

All faiths and systems of religious belief and practice constitute
various rituals, rules and systems of spiritual practice designed to
help an individual find and deepen their inner life and connection with
God or spirit.

Some knowledge of others' beliefs and religious practice can help the primary
care team develop practice that is sensitive to the patient's deepest needs.
However, it is not enough to simply label a patient 'Church of England' or
'Buddhist' and make assumptions about his or her needs. The doctor or nurse
needs an awareness of the variations between faiths, within faiths and between
the people who follow those faiths.

21.1 Interfaith variation

General information about some of the main faith groups in the UK is given
below. By necessity this is a simplification!

21.2 Intrafaith variation

Within each faith group are subgroups, which may have important differences
in practice. For example, a Buddhist may follow the Tibetan, Therevada or
Zen traditions. Tibetan Buddhism is devotional and colourful; Zen Buddhism
intellectual and austere. In Judaism there are many differences in belief and
practice between a strictly orthodox Jew, who will usually wish a burial as
quickly as possible, not leaving the body unattended in the meantime, and a
liberal Reform Jew, who may be quite happy with a post-mortem and may even
carry an organ donor card.

Within the Christian tradition, there is likewise no place for assumption or complacency. A Roman Catholic may wish candles, a rosary, the blessing of the sick (a sacramental ritual better known to lay-people as the 'last rites') and various devotional icons or medallions. A Quaker whose worship is in a shared silence waiting on the word of God within, may simply wish to share that silence with other members of the 'meeting'. A Jehovah's witness may have a literal interpretation of scriptural passages, which alters the acceptability of blood and blood products intravenously.

21.3 Inter-individual variation

All religions are a balance of the outer form (the external) with the inner journey of that individual person (the internal). The outer form is easily visible, even to people of no religious belief, with attendance at services, participation in rituals and so on. The inner journey may only be apparent in deep conversation, or in the unfolding of a response to a difficult situation. This can confuse the health worker who may assume that a regular churchgoer will automatically have deep spiritual reserves to call upon.

One woman regarded herself as Christian, but rarely went to church or read the Bible. However, she experienced a deep sense of the closeness of God and believed no matter what happened she would be given the strength to face it. This sense grew, as she became more ill. Another woman, similar in age, had been a 'pillar' of the local church. She could not believe it when her cancer was diagnosed, and saw it as a punishment for some wrongdoing by a punitive God. She experienced a major crisis in her faith.

Individual people (as well as different faiths or sects) will vary in how much relative importance is given to the inner journey or the outer form. For most people, the outer form of the faith connects and supports the inner journey, and faith practice is a source of strength, growth and love. However occasionally, the outer form is practised dogmatically, with little or no connection with an inner spiritual journey, and this can increase fear and rigidity when a crisis comes (*Figure 21.3.1*).

Different people, even within one subgroup of one faith, will vary in many ways. Some may put a greater emphasis on one aspect of practice or be strict about one particular rule; others may have little concern about rules, placing great store on the experience of the presence of God.

However involved in faith practice an individual has been, serious illness and impending death raise many fundamental questions, and beliefs are revisited at a deeper level. Often this leads to a deepening of faith and understanding, but occasionally it leads to a loss of a belief that may have been held since childhood. This can be painful, and a source of great suffering. The following chapter, *Chapter 22: spiritual care in a secular society*, may help in supporting this sort of situation.

Inner journey		Outer form
Direct sense of transcendence	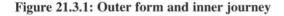	Rituals, rules, practice
Inner connection with God or spirit		System of beliefs
Flexibility		Rigidity
Growth		Dogma
Love		Fear

Figure 21.3.1: Outer form and inner journey

The guidance that follows is of necessity very general (*Table 21.3.1*).

A good practice will form links with key members of its local cultural and faith groups. It will carry a list of faith leaders or advisers and their contact details. Most importantly, it will ask patient and family what is right for them, it will listen with sensitivity, openness and acceptance to the reply and it will endeavour to ensure that healthcare practice is flexible enough to adapt to the cultural or religious needs of that patient and family.

Areas to ask about are:

- specific dietary restrictions
- sacred festivals
- washing and personal care
- modesty/gender rules for personal care and medical examination
- rituals and beliefs about care while dying
- rituals and beliefs about care after death.

In general, Asian patients are much more modest in dress and behaviour than Westerners. This applies particularly to women, who may be acutely embarrassed or distressed if medical or nursing care is not sensitive to these needs, which may include a need for care from a same-sex health worker.

Standards of cleanliness are often high, and sitting in a bath may be regarded as unclean. Running water or a shower is preferred for washing, which may be frequent. The left hand may be regarded as 'unclean', being used for washing after using the toilet. Touching someone with the left hand with this cultural practice is regarded as offensive.

Table 21.1.1: Spiritual care pack © Eileen Palmer, 2004

Faith	Diet	Sacred festivals	Washing	Modesty	Care while dying	Care after death
Buddhism (Buddhist monk, lay teacher or lama for Tibetan Buddhism) More information from: www.buddhanet.net	Often vegetarian. May avoid alcohol/mind altering drugs. Vesak (Buddha day) May	Buddhist New Year Jan, Feb or April depending on country of origin. Puja days (days of festival/prayer linked to lunar cycle) Vesak (Buddha day) May	No special needs	Variable needs. Asians may prefer same gender doctor/nurse	Important to die consciously with a clear mind. May refuse painkillers/sedatives. Prefer to know they are dying. May wish a Buddhist monk to be present, but not many other visitors	Believe consciousness remains in the body 8–12 hours. May not wish the body to be touched too soon. Chanting from the Abhidhamma (Theravada) or Tibetan book of the Dead (Tibetan). Rituals and practice vary — check with family. Cremation common
Christianity Religious leader: priest, vicar, elder More information from: www.geneva.rutgers.edu/src/christianity	No special needs. Some abstain from a favourite food during Lent. Sometimes abstain from meat on Fridays/fast before communion	Holy day is Sunday (Saturday for Seventh Day Adventists) Advent (Dec 1–24); Christmas (25 Dec); Lent (40 days up to Easter); Easter (March/April calculated by lunar calendar); Whitsun or Pentecost (50 days after Easter)	No special needs (check for cultural preference)	No special needs	Sacrament of the sick/'last rites' may be important for Roman Catholics and some Anglicans. Prayers and communion may be welcomed. Other practices vary — check with patient, family and faith community	Body treated with respect and dignity. Support from clergy as required. May wish to pray. No formal problems with postmortem. Usually church funeral followed by burial or cremation. (Requiem mass for Catholics)

Table 21.1.1: Spiritual care pack © Eileen Palmer, 2004

Hinduism Religious leader: Brahmin priest or pandit More information: www.hinduism.co.za	Often vegetarian. Ban on beef Fasting common	Divali (Festival of lights) Oct/Nov calculated by lunar calendar; Sankrantis 12 solar festivals; Vasant Panchami Spring festival; Navaratri (9 nights); and Dassera (Mother goddess) Holi (March). Many others celebrating Hindu Gods	Wash daily in running water. Wash hands and mouth with water before/after food. Total privacy for bedbaths. Wash private parts with running water after excretion	Women often require female doctor/nurse. Men may request male nurse for personal care	Prefer to die at home. Atonement ceremony with Brahmin priest at home, may be followed by blessing and tying of sacred thread around the wrist. (Do not remove these threads.) Family/extended family brings gifts for the patient to touch for distribution to the needy. Sacred leaves and Ganges water may be placed in the mouth before death. May wish to die on the floor, close to Mother Earth	Body left uncovered. Consult the family before touching the body. Family usually do Last Rites, washing patient with sacred water. Postmortem only for legal requirement. All organs to be returned. Funeral preferred within 24 hours. Always cremation. Eldest son is chief mourner; women may stay at home
Islam Religious leader: Imam or maulana More information: www.islam.com	Ban on pork and alcohol. Ban on non-Halal meat, often vegetarian. Fast between sunrise and sunset for a month at Ramadam (partial/total exceptions for elderly or ill)	Muslim holy day is Friday Jum'a-tul-Mubarak (Friday prayer) Ramadan lasts one month (variable calculated by lunar calendar); Eid-ul-Fitr end of Ramadan; Eid-al-Adha (April); Muharram Eid Milad-un-Nabi Shab-i-Miraj; Lailat-ul-Qadr	Wash daily in running water. Wash before prayers. Women wash completely after menstruation. Wash private parts with running water after excretion	Crucial for men and women. Women clothed head to foot day and night. Women need female doctors/nurses	May wish to face Mecca (SE in the UK) Family may recite Koran Family will probably wish to stay with the patient and may wish an Iman to be present. Children often actively excluded from death and after-death rituals/ceremonies	Do **not** wash the body, cut nails or hair. Non-Muslim should not touch body. Wear gloves if vital to touch. Mosque or family will handle ritual washing of the body and prayers. Postmortem only if legal requirement — organs to be buried with the body. Burial (never cremation), within 24 hours performed only by men

Table 21.1.1: Spiritual care pack © Eileen Palmer, 2004

Judaism Religious leader: Rabbi More information: www.jewish. co.uk	'Kosher' diet. No pork or shellfish. Kosher meat. No mixing of meat and milk (even in food preparation)	Jewish Sabbath sundown on Friday until sundown on Saturday Pesach (Passover) April; Shavot June (49 days after Pesach); Rosh Hashanah (Jewish New Year) Sept/Oct; Yom Kippur (atonement)	No special needs	No special needs generally. Ultra- orthodox Jews may wish to keep hair and limbs covered. Men may regard physical contact from female staff as immodest.	Dying patient is not left alone, family will usually want to be present at death. Prayers recited by relatives. May require Rabbi (ask family)	Allow time lapse before touching body and touch as little as possible. Arms extended by sides with hands open. Do not wash the body. Ritual purification by Holy Assembly. Postmortem only for legal requirement. Burial within 24 hours apart from Sabbath. Cremation forbidden
Sikhs Religious leader: Sikh community More information: www. gurudwaras.org	Often vegetarian. Ban on Halal meat and alcohol. May avoid beef and/or pork	Baisakhi (April); Gurpurab (10 per year, celebrating the 10 gurus of the Khalsa Panth); Prakash Utsav (festival of light); Holla Mohalla (festival of colour and happiness)	Wash daily in running water. Wash hands and mouth with water before/ after food. Wash private parts with running water after excretion	Female doctor/ nurse for female patients if possible. The Kaccha (undershorts) is a sacred garment. Consult closely with patient if it needs removing	Family may wish to sing or say prayers. The 5 Ks are personal sacred objects, not to be removed Kesh: uncut hair Kanga: wooden comb, fixing the hair Kara: metal wristband on the right wrist Kaccha: underpants Kirpan: dagger	Body may be laid on the floor Continue special regard for 5 Ks Family may wish to wash the body. Viewing important No formal problems with postmortem Always cremated as soon as possible (within 24 hours)

Carers don't have an idea about cultural diversity — but they only need to listen for a few moments to be sensitive.

Sikh doctor (Firth, 1993)

Key points

❖ There is variability between faiths, within faiths and between members of any one faith.

❖ A good practice will form links with key members and advisers from local faith and cultural groups to act as a resource.

❖ If in doubt, ask the patient and family rather than assume.

❖ Religious practice does not always correlate with inner spiritual resource, and this applies to any faith.

References

Firth S (1993) Death in Hindu and Sikh communities. In: Dickenson D, Johnson M, eds. *Death, Dying and Bereavement*. Sage Publications, London: 244–61

Further reading

Neuberger J (2003) *Caring for Dying People of Different Faiths*. 3rd edn. Radcliffe Medical Press, Oxford

Rees D (1997) *Death and Bereavement: the Psychological, Religious and Cultural Interfaces*. Whurr publishers, London

Murray Parkes C, Laungani P, Young B (1997) *Death and Bereavement Across Cultures*. Routledge, London and New York

22

Spiritual care in a secular society

Birth is a miracle, death is a mystery; neither fits neatly with the biomedical model....

22.1 What is spirituality?

As doctors and nurses we are well trained in a biomedical, problem-solving model of care. This leads us to focus on the concrete, the measurable and use experience, for example on the relief of pain or other symptoms. We are not so well trained, and indeed can often feel most out of our depth, when faced with spiritual needs, which rarely lend themselves to a simple problem-solving approach.

Spirituality is defined by what we are, rather than what we do. Many definitions abound. A recent conference on spirituality in palliative care summarized the essence of these.

> *Spirituality is that faculty present in all human beings that causes them to search for meaning in what is happening to them, to attempt to make sense for themselves of the world as they perceive it, and to draw conclusions/beliefs from their own observations that shape their behaviour. This power or life-force (spirit or soul in the language of religion) has the potential to create invisible resources to sustain, motivate and transform the way in which an individual experiences his or her life.*

Dufour, 2000

From this definition, spiritual care is care that encourages and supports reflection on experience, the search for meaning and the development of inner resources for the journey.

Physical care needs to work in harmony with the spiritual care. Are we helping the patient in his or her journey and development of inner resources, or are we inadvertently undermining them? It is easy to step in with our own beliefs and biomedical models and to believe these are the only truth.

Our spirituality is akin to the whole of our inner journey, not only through cancer or a serious illness, but also through the whole of our individual and unique life experience. Its starts with the unique alive spark that is one human being. It travels through the inner journey that is one human life with its loves, its passions, its hardships, its monotony and its pain. Within that it forges relationships, both good and bad, it feels, it suffers, it laughs, it is moved to tears or it trembles with joy. It contains strength, inspiration and vision. It contains vulnerability, doubt and fear. When it is at its best, it allows us to grow, to transcend suffering, to find meaning, to move on, to inspire or uplift others. When it is struggling, it may leave us frightened, trapped and tormented by fear, bitterness, cynicism or hopelessness.

22.2 Spirituality and religion

Spirituality and religion are often confused and sometimes used as interchangeable words; they are not. A religion is a belief system, often linked with rituals and practices, which may help many people to better spiritual understanding by giving a framework for their experience.

An analogy Jean Radley (2002) (district nurse and Anglican priest) uses is that spirituality is like a hand, something everyone has, an integral part of the human form. Some people may find a glove into which the hand comfortably fits, and this glove is religion. Other people may choose to forgo the glove, yet they will still have the spiritual part of themselves. Others may choose a glove with a poor fit, or even one that does not fit at all, but looks like the neighbour's gloves.

Thus we can sometimes meet people who are regular churchgoers who may have great difficulty and immense spiritual pain. Someone else with no particular religious affiliation or faith may face a terrible situation with immense courage and inner resource, inspiring all around them.

22.3 What are spiritual needs?

All of us — doctors, nurses, other team members, patients and carers — will have spiritual needs. All spiritual needs are derived from two core needs; the need for love and the need to find meaning.

The need for love/positive regard

The core spiritual need is to love and to be loved, to be accepted for who or what we are. A powerful and poignant example of this was what we know of the experience of those caught up in the aeroplane hijackings of 11 September 2001. Every message in the face of impending death was to a loved one to affirm that love. Good spiritual care means love, unconditional positive regard for the person in front of us. In many faiths, God or spirit is described as love. Service given to others has been described as 'love in action'. As such all healthcare workers could be regarded as providing spiritual care.

This need for love is not always expressed through relationships with others. It can also be expressed through a relationship with a transcendent force, with God or spirit, through a love of the earth or of the natural world. It may be expressed through a love of music, art, poetry, gardening, a pet, a huge richness of things that over the centuries have made up the diversity and vastness of the human spirit. Many people, even in our urban Western societies, are immeasurably moved by the dawn or the sunset, the stars at night, the waves of the ocean or the flow of a river. These things may become even more important as a patient approaches death.

The need for meaning

He who has a 'why' to live for can bear almost any 'how'.

Friedrich Nietzshe, 1844–1900

The second spiritual need is the need for meaning, for purpose in life. The search for meaning is deep in humanity. Viktor Frankl was a psychiatrist who spent three years suffering unimaginable physical and emotional horror in concentration camps in Auschwitz and Dachau. He described how suffering even in this extreme situation could be transformed by the power of the individual to give it meaning. 'Everything can be taken from a man but one thing: the last of the human freedoms — to choose one's attitude in any given set of circumstances.' He describes how vital this was for the inmates' very survival and sense of self to believe their suffering had meaning. His personal journey was to a realization of love as the ultimate and highest goal of humankind — even more extraordinary when we try to imagine the horror and cruelty of his daily existence at that time.

Many doctors and nurses are continually humbled by the spirit of patients faced with serious illness — their humour, their concern for their families, even for their health carers. The search for meaning may be expressed in many ways. It may come out as questions such as 'Why me?' or 'What have I done to deserve this?' There may be a need to review the past, to talk about what happened when and why. Some will turn to religion, maybe in a different or deeper way. Both within and outside of organized religions, many will review their relationship with God, the beliefs of their childhood and ways they have touched the transcendant and eternal. Many will look at their life as it is with an urgent sense of what means most to them, and seek to deepen, nurture or repair the most important relationships that surround them. Maybe there will be an important journey still to make or a holiday to leave a legacy of shared memories and closeness. Others may join or even found support groups for patients with a similar illness, or raise funds for a local healthcare charity.

> *The impulse is deep in human beings to seek to transform pain and suffering, not by denying it, but by feeling it in the depths of our being and giving it meaning.*
>
> Hermann Hesse, 1877–1962

From these two basic needs, other spiritual needs arise (see *Figure 22.3.1*).

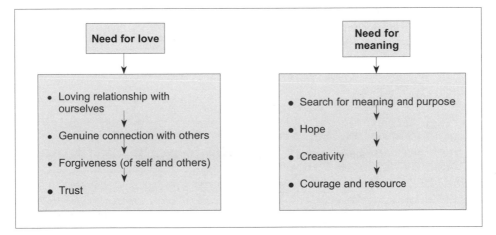

Figure 22.3.1: Spirituality, love and meaning

As healthcare workers we need to be able to support this basic process, and also to recognize when it is going wrong and spiritual pain is present.

22.4 Does spiritual care matter?

A study from Sweden showed meaningfulness to be the item with the strongest correlation to global quality of life for both patients and spouses with incurable cancer. A questionnaire to 1426 doctors, carers, seriously ill patients and recently bereaved family members showed that patients consistently place much higher value on emotional and spiritual aspects of care than their doctors did (*Table 22.4.1*) (Steinhauser, 2000).

The relative importance of spiritual aspects of care grows with the seriousness of the illness and the impact on the patient's beliefs about his or her life expectancy (*Figure 22.4.1*).

Table 22.4.1: Results of survey assessing the value of different aspects of care

Important attribute of care	Patients	Doctors
Being mentally aware	92%	65%
Being at peace with God	89%	65%
Being able to pray	85%	55%
Feeling one's life is complete	80%	68%

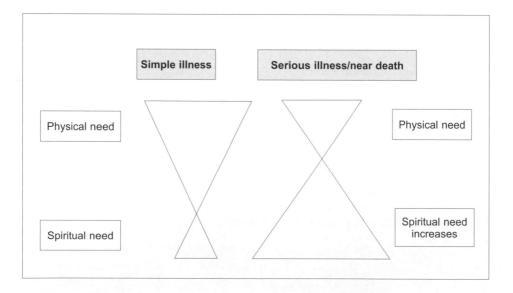

Figure 22.4.1: The increase in spiritual need as death approaches

22.5 What is spiritual pain?

Spiritual pain arises when there is a gap between a person's innermost sense of value and meaning and the external reality. It is a deep pain. It threatens the integrity of the whole person — life falls apart or seems utterly meaningless, devoid of all hope. To use religious language it is a 'dark night of the soul'. This pain can be experienced as real suffering and anguish. It can make physical symptoms almost impossible to address (*Figure 22.5.1*).

Our inner sense of who we are is based on decades of lived experience, expectation and deeply ingrained habit. We all hope to live to see our grandchildren. We all assume cancer happens to someone else, not us. An event such as a serious illness challenges all of this. It challenges our beliefs about life, about ourselves and about the future. It challenges our inner sense of meaning. Somehow, painfully, we have to let go of everything we thought 'ought to be' and enter a separation, adjustment or grief reaction. Some individuals may have an inner life, a spiritual self that allows them to adjust easily to this.

> David was forty-seven years with established paralysis of his lower body from a lung cancer that had caused spread into his thoracic vertebrae causing spinal cord compression. He said 'I know there's no betterment and I know where this is leading, but I'm forty-seven and I feel I've had a good innings. I've done what mattered for me.'

For others there is a painful journey as they let go of deeply held beliefs. They travel a dark and difficult path, a 'dark night of the soul', with familiar securities and survival skills overwhelmed by confusion, anguish, and 'a terrible fatigue of the spirit'. Gradually, they may come to a new and different sense of things, they may find a meaning that is utterly different to anything they had previously believed, but that allows them to make sense of things, to move on, and a peace comes again.

> Agnes was eighty years and had battled with cancer for years. Despite this she found the diagnosis of a new primary lymphoma unbearable. She was overwhelmed by fear and anxiety, telephoning her GP and family members frequently in deep distress. She was convinced she must have done something terrible at some stage in her life and that God was punishing her for leaving an abusive marriage some years previously. Although she had much care and support, she struggled through most of her last months to make sense of what was happening or why. She continued to express a lot of guilt. It was difficult to sense any progress, but the support continued. In her last weeks she had a series of meaningful conversations with her son, and was able to come to a sense of self-forgiveness and real peace.

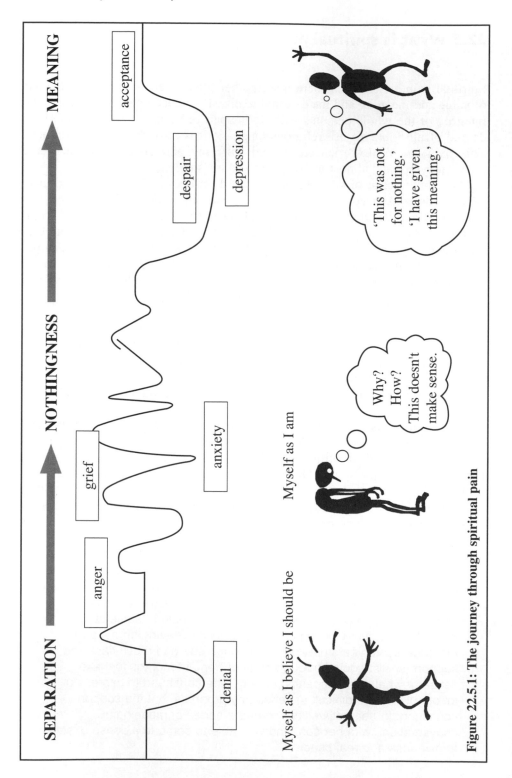

Figure 22.5.1: The journey through spiritual pain

22.6 Symptoms of spiritual pain

Love and meaning have been described above as core spiritual needs for all people from which other needs derive. The symptoms of spiritual pain are derived from a lack of love and a loss of meaning. This manifests as in *Figure 22.6.1.*

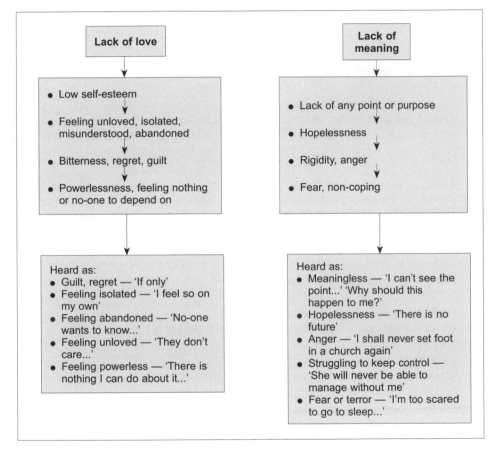

Figure 22.6.1: Symptoms of spiritual pain

Fear of dying is widespread and deep. It may reflect many aspects of the above process. Seven common fears of dying have been described:

⌘ Fear of the dying process — 'What will it be like?' 'Will it be painful?'
⌘ Fear of loss of control — 'Will I be dependant on others?' 'Will I be unable to care for myself?'
⌘ Fear of loss of loved ones — 'How will they manage without me?'

⌘ Fear of others' reaction to them — 'How will people cope with seeing me like this?'
⌘ Fear of isolation — 'Will people stop coming to see me?'
⌘ Fear of the unknown — 'What happens after you die?'
⌘ Fear that life will have been meaningless.

Naming and recognizing the fear can reduce it.

22.6 Helping someone with spiritual pain

This can seem one of the most difficult and challenging areas of care, and one for which there is little training. It involves a shift from our usual behaviour patterns of doing, problem solving, generating solutions to being, knowing we have no answers and living with life's questions and uncertainties.

There is good evidence that the degree to which healthcare professionals can recognize or respond to spiritual need relates to their ability to do this for themselves. A healthcare worker who is not comfortable with a sense of man (or woman) as a spiritual being is less likely to recognize spiritual need and less likely to refer. It is worthwhile ensuring the team has at least one member who is comfortable with the concept and recognition of spiritual need.

Providing spiritual care means:

- working with love/positive regard
- encouraging and supporting the search for meaning
- fostering hope
- understanding loss and grief
- allowing expression of emotional and spiritual needs
- involving chaplains and spiritual care workers
- meeting our own spiritual needs.

I meet one of the GPs and say to him 'I have breast cancer'. What does it feel like to say the words out loud? He listens as I pour out my feelings and is very gentle. Talking has helped.

I meet my own GP. He also listens sympathetically, and this time I cry. He gives no false promises — I wouldn't want him to — above all I want everyone to be honest with me. But he does give me hope — and right now I need that more than anything else.

Woman with breast cancer

Working with love/positive regard

In practical terms this means the following.

Being genuine. Being ourselves, communicating with honesty and integrity. Not being afraid to 'not have all the answers'. Being courageous enough to acknowledge our powerlessness, the gaps in what we can offer and do. Remembering that as well as our professional role we are also another human being, on the same journey, albeit at a different point.

Respecting the patient's individuality. Respecting who a patient is, this unique life in front of us, that has never been before, that will never be repeated and allowing him or her to 'do it in his or her own way'. Generally, the way people have approached their life will determine the way they approach their dying. Recognize this; encourage the use of what works for them, even if you think you would choose to do it differently.

Deep listening. A lot of medical and nursing listening is selective, and aimed at pattern recognition and problem solving. It is characterized by focussed and closed questions (giving yes/no or right/wrong answers) to allow the doctor or nurse to choose the 'right' course of action. Deep listening is a different skill. The only goal of this sort of listening is understanding. To really understand the person in front of us, we need to let go of what we think we know and listen deeply. Deep listening is listening without prejudice; listening without assumption, judgment or solution. It is much more about hearing the question, than giving the answer, properly hearing the question in the depth of our being. It assumes the patient has the power to find his or her own answers (if any exist) within him/herself, and our role is to facilitate this and to witness it. Dame Cicely Saunders calls this 'The need for a listener' and 'sharing in the silence'.

Skills of deep listening:

⌘ Attentive silence (keeping the mouth shut and the ears open) allows the patient to explore his or her inner world without judgment or comment. Just listen.
⌘ To listen with the whole of our being. To sit and be present. If the patient is stuck, additional skills such as paraphrasing, reflecting feelings or the echoing of key words or phrases may help, but should not be used to intrude on natural periods of silent reflection.
⌘ We should avoid giving 'answers' or burdening the patient with our own beliefs or expectations, such as 'you will find peace comes' or 'God will take care of you' or even 'speak to the chaplain and you will feel much better'. This can close down communication. It can also leave a patient doubly burdened, feeling as though he or she has somehow failed if

peace or ease is not found. Sometimes, even with best care, a patient may struggle to let go.

Do not go gentle into that good night.
Old age should burn and rave at close of day.
Rage, rage against the dying of the light.

Dylan Thomas, 1914–1953

⌘ Expressing empathy, warmth and positive regard. Basic human warmth and a kind, attentive silence allow a safe space to open where pain and suffering can be faced, and transformed gradually into peace and acceptance. This can sometimes seem a great challenge, and a low priority in a busy day, but it stems naturally from even short periods of deep listening.

Encouraging and supporting the search for meaning

There are many ways to find meaning, such as:

- through existing belief, faith or spiritual practice
- in the network of friendship and companionship built up over a lifetime
- starting a spiritual practice, such as meditation. This is a simple way to inner stillness and a sense of inner peace and connection, which requires no belief system
- creative therapies or any activity the patient can draw inspiration from. Sometimes this can include a reconnection with hobbies from childhood or young adult life
- complementary therapies
- reading inspirational books, listening to music
- sharing with others who have suffered in different ways.

A useful working framework is the '4 Rs', described in *A Handbook for Mortals* by Dr Joanne Lynn and Dr Joan Harrold (1999).

Remembering. Remembering and re-telling important parts of the life story. This can be as simple as asking about important relationships ('How long have you been together?' 'How did you meet?') or photographs in the room. The patient/family might be encouraged to look through a photograph album. Writing, artwork, making a photographic collage or a video- or audiotape can be more formal methods of life review. Keeping a journal or diary can help. The story is not just the medical story, but what has mattered for the patient.

Reassessing. Remembering and re-telling events can allow a re-evaluation of their significance and reflection on how and why a particular course of action was taken. This may be a simple process ('I was younger then, and just didn't know any better...') or something more complex.

Reconciling. The processes of remembering and reassessing important events can sometimes allow a space to develop for reconciliation. This is an acceptance of what happened and why, an acceptance of imperfections and a true forgiveness of self and others if blame and hurt are still present.

Reuniting. Coming to a sense of inner peace can then help a coming together with family members or friends who have been estranged or distant. Sometimes, there may be a re-uniting with a religious life that had been discarded.

> He couldn't even grasp my hand, but he was tapping it with his finger to reassure me he knew what I was saying. You know they say when people are leaving the world, they see a light, I don't know what it was he saw, although his eyes were focused on me at the point of death he looked up, and this most wonderful expression came across his face, like he was looking at something really magical. He was just like a child looking at something new and fabulous they have been given as a gift. He just had this look of amazement on his face and he looked like he was being drawn towards something. He died with this peaceful, amazing look on his face because at that point he closed his eyes and he was gone.
> It was a moving experience, but very significant for me because it really did look as if God had come to collect him. The look on his face always comforts me; even though my sleep is invaded each night with images of him in different stages of his illness, I still can't believe how rapidly and devastatingly this cancer took hold of him.

Wife describing the death of her husband who had been frightened by his diagnosis and had struggled to come to terms with it.

Fostering hope

Hope is the deep nourishment that keeps the human soul going, despite everything. This goes so far that Elizabeth Kübler-Ross (1979), from her observations of many dying patients in her seminal work *On Death and Dying* made the observation that, 'when a patient stops expressing hope it is a sign of imminent death'. Hope is very different to optimism or positive thinking. The latter, may ignore or deny the negative. Hope embraces the negative, but still hopes, for a few days longer, for a miracle cure, for a peaceful death, for life to have meant something.

The counterpart of hope is emptiness or even despair. Good doctors and nurses will never underestimate the importance of hope; the spirit that allows men or women to survive war, natural disaster, concentration camps against all the evidence to the contrary. It is easy to confuse hope with denial. In reality patients can be fully aware of their predicament, but still choose to hope for the best, at least some of the time.

Hope is fostered, not by untruth but by:

- gentle truth telling
- respectful relationship
- realistic goals.

Understanding loss and grief

To understand loss and grief we need to understand the nature of normal adjustment reactions, the inner journey, the experience of transition and the human responses to loss and grief. The more we can understand these parts of what it is to be human, the more we are able to be with suffering, rather than withdrawing from the things we feel we cannot 'fix'.

Allowing expression of emotional and spiritual needs

This usually means giving the patient permission to express his or her needs at this level. The simplest way to do this is to ask about any emotional or spiritual concerns and be prepared to listen to the answer. For example, 'How are you, with everything that's been happening?' 'How are you feeling?'

Involving chaplains and spiritual care workers

Chaplains and others regularly involved in delivering spiritual care have expertise we can draw from. They can provide a different 'non-health' perspective that can broaden our vision and approach to issues around death and dying. They can offer skill in one-to-one work with patients with spiritual pain.

Like many specialist services:

- they are often involved too late
- their involvement needs sensitive negotiation
- they can support and help develop skills of team members, even where their direct involvement is inappropriate.

As well as faith-based ministers or chaplains, new disciplines such as 'interfaith' ministry are developing, which may be more responsive to the diversity of spiritual and religious need in contemporary society.

Meeting our own spiritual needs

This work is only possible if we are able to recognize and meet our own needs. Healthcare professionals also suffer with palliative care. A Polish study of eighty-one GPs (Luczak, 1999) found that in dealing with terminal illness, GPs reported: suffering (86%); sadness (90%); helplessness (89%); and powerlessness (85%).

To continue to care we need to care for ourselves. This can involve some or all of the following:

- sharing and support from within the practice team/close confidant/skilled supervisor/mentor/counsellor
- reflective practice
- improving our communication skills
- acknowledging our limits
- setting sustainable boundaries between work and home life
- finding sources of love/positive regard and meaningful activity in our own lives
- deepening our intimate relationships
- creativity
- spending time in nature
- deepening a faith or belief that sustains us
- finding a regular spiritual practice (such as meditation, which can reduce anxiety and improve inner well-being)
- develop emotional insight through personal development work, coaching, mentoring, Balint groups, support groups
- reviewing the role of money in our lives.

Seeking occupational prestige or a high income are strongly associated with misery!

When we are finally forced to confront our own powerlessness in the face of death, we can increasingly come to practice a different, humbler but stronger form of medicine; a medicine of the heart and the soul. We do this when we sit, not as doctor or nurse and patient, but as one mortal human being with another, listening with our hearts open to the experience of the person we are with.

*The primary thing he and I needed is kindness. When you are
dealing with the most shocking thing of your life, it just blows you*

away. You don't want to hear anything less than kind. I know the doctor is busy, but there is no way you want to feel 'Right, you've had your five minutes or your ten minutes now, you must go.'

You want to feel that at this time in his life, he means everything. The care they are providing, they need to reassure the patient that everything possible is being done. When, with good reason, the nurse came on a different day, he got quite upset, because he was so insecure and knocked sideways. The reassurance and the care are the most needed thing of a cancer patient. Kindness and empathy, and absolutely no way should they be treated 'Oh well, you are terminally ill, it doesn't matter'; that's my theory anyway.

Wife of patient with lung cancer

A qualitative study of 130 primary-care doctors in Wisconsin, USA (Yamey and Wilkes, 2001), showed the five main methods of sustaining well-being were:

❖ Time with family and friends.
❖ Religious/spiritual activity.
❖ Self-care.
❖ Finding meaning in work *and* setting boundaries around it.
❖ Philosophical outlook, such as positive thinking/focusing on success.

Key points

❖ Spirituality and religion are different things.
❖ Core spiritual needs derive from the need for love and the need for meaning.
❖ Spiritual pain arises from a lack of love or meaning. It can present with a range of symptoms.
❖ Patients attach more importance to spiritual wellbeing than doctors.
❖ Kindness, compassion and deep listening are core skills.
❖ To care for our patients, we need good mechanisms of caring for ourselves.
❖ Hope is fostered not by untruth but by gentle truth telling, respect and realistic goals.

References

Dufour P (2000) Spirituality in Palliative Care. Conference of Association of Hospice Chaplains, Trinity Hospice, London

Frankl VE (1959) Man's Search for Meaning. Beacon Press, Washington Square Press

Kübler-Ross E (1979) *On Death and Dying*. Tavistock, London

Luczak J (1999) Medical obligation to beat suffering. VI Congress of the European Association for Palliative Care, Geneva

Lynn J, Harrold J (1999) A *Handbook for Mortals; Guidance for People Facing Serious Illness*. Oxford University Press, Oxford

Steinhauser KE, Christakis NA, Clipp EC, McNeilly M, McIntyre L, Tulsky JA (2000) Factors considered important at the end of life by patients, family, physicians and other care providers. *JAMA* **284**(19): 2476–82

Yamey G, Wilkes M (2001) Promoting wellbeing among doctors. *Br Med J* 322: 252–3

Further reading

Callananm, Kelly P (1992) *Final Gifts: Understanding and helping the dying*. Hodder and Stoughton, London

Cole R (1997) Meditation in palliative care — a practical tool for self-management. *Palliative Med* **11**: 411–13

Edassery D, Kuttierath SK (1998) Spirituality in the secular sense. *Eur J Palliative Care* **5**: 165–7

Freeman L (1996) A short span of days: meditation and care for the dying patient, family and caregiver. Transcript of talks to teh 7th International Congress on Palliative Care, Novalis/Medio Media, Montreal

Hamilton Rev DG (1998) Believing in patient's beliefs: physician attunement to the spiritual dimension as a positive factor in patient healing and health. *Am J Hospice Palliative Care*: Sept/Oct

Hegarty M (2001) The dynamic of hope: hoping in the face of death. *Progress Palliative Care* **9**: 42–6

Kearney M (1996) *Mortally Wounded*. Marino, Dublin

King M, Speck P, Thomas A (1999) The effect of spiritual beliefs on outcome from illness. *Soc Sci Med* **48**: 1291–99

McCabe MJ (1997) Clinical response to spiritual issues. In: Portenoy RK, Bruera E, eds. *Topics in Palliative Care*. Oxford University Press, Oxford:

McClain CS, Rosenfeld B, Breitbart W (2003) Effect of spiritual wellbeing on end of life despair in terminally ill cancer patients. *Lancet* **361**: 1603–7

23

Grief, mourning and bereavement

*I was scared all the time of everything going wrong, because I had
never had to worry about a thing; he was this brilliant man who
fixed everything, sorted everything. I never even used to worry about
locking the doors last thing at night because he did all that sort of
thing. He even fed the cats last thing at night and covered the budgie
up. Suddenly all these creatures to care for were my responsibility
alone. It was pretty scary.*

*Because it was such a scary thing, my immediate family didn't
always know what to say. Yet I needed to hear it, to hear words of
comfort, words of encouragement. I was so totally lost without him,
I didn't even know if I could carry on without him. I know you hear
people say that, but I truly did believe it; I couldn't live without him.*

Bereaved woman, aged fifty

Bereavement

Bereavement, the loss of someone dearly loved, is one the most painful human
experiences. The process by which it is travelled through is called grief. It is
said that grief starts when the illness is diagnosed, and both patient and family
face a whole series of griefs or losses. This section deals with bereavement; the
experience of the survivors.

Grief is associated with increased rates of both physical and mental illness,
and increased mortality. Most cultures and societies have customs, rituals
and ways of marking bereavement and the grieving process. This is called
mourning. It is designed to support the bereaved person through the grieving
process. Mourning rituals are largely absent in contemporary British society.
This can be a real problem, when friends or work colleagues may expect the
bereaved person to be 'over it' a few weeks after a major loss.

I was shocked when a good friend, who was also a healthcare
worker, asked me 'Why are you upset?' 'I still miss him all the
time' I said. It was six weeks since his death, and I was in complete
turmoil. 'Haven't you got over that yet?' she asked incredulously.

Bereaved healthcare worker

The common misconceptions about grief are:

⌘ That people 'get over it' quickly. Significant loss produces grief of
significant duration. Many people describe taking several years to adjust
to a major loss, sometimes longer.
⌘ That the bereaved person will 'return to normal'. The truth is that the
bereaved person will be forever changed. People who have experienced
significant loss speak of 'never being the same again'.

Recovery from grief is marked by the ability to re-engage with life again. The
loss is assimilated, the experience becomes a part of the individual's life story
and they are different, but able to continue with life in a rewarding way. Like
childbirth, the experience is not forgotten — it remains vivid. Even many years
later, widowed people will describe an inner sense of relationship with the dead
person that can manifest in a comforting sense of their presence at times. Their
eyes may still fill when they recall a loss. They may still experience auditory
or visual hallucinations of the deceased person, especially after an unusually
long or close relationship.

23.1 Normal grief

Like all adjustment reactions, grief moves through a series of stages, although it
can seem quite overwhelming at the outset. These are not necessarily followed
in a linear way. People may seem to skip a stage, move forwards or backwards.
Sometimes an individual will get stuck in a particular stage and seem unable
to move on (*Table 23.1.1*).

However hard it is to see or imagine, this sense of a progression, an
underlying journey, a distant light, can sometimes help the bereaved person.

What he said was encouraging. He drew a little diagram of a heart
— I always remembered that. The heart was all black and he said,
'at first this is what it is like. Your heart is so leadened with the grief
there's no brightness on the horizon at all. After several months you
will start to feel better, and a little corner of that heart will start to
let a chink of light in, you start to become interested in something

again. You will maybe take an interest in a bit of your garden, you will take a social gathering up and, sometime after that, more light will appear in the darkness of your heart because you will realize you are moving on. That may not happen for many months to come, but I can assure you it will get better.

Bereaved woman describing a supportive intervention

Grief may vary in time course and in intensity or depth. Generally, variants in the progression of grief are because of avoidance of facing and working through the pain of the loss.

The grieving process is described diagramatically in *Figure 23.1.1*.

Table 23.1.1: Stages of grief

Stage (and other terms)	Duration (variable)	Common experiences	Underlying task
Early (initial reactions)	Days to weeks (0–28 days)	Numbness Shock Disbelief	'The loss' Accepting the reality of the loss
Middle (acute mourning, acute grief)	Months (6–12 months)	Anger, guilt Yearning, pining Restless searching Sense or hallucination of the dead person's presence (50%) Anxiety, agitation, panic Physical symptoms: loss of appetite, sleep disturbance, fatigue, exhaustion Loneliness, isolation Depression, despair, desolation Apathy	'Separation and nothingness' Working through the pain of grief
Late (resolution, adaptation)	Years (6–12 months to 2–5 years)	Sadness Sense of emptiness within Re-engaging with life, with interests, with friends Developing a new sense of meaning Coming to terms with the loss Healing: sense of inner growth, deeper understanding/compassion	'Integration and finding meaning' Adjusting to the new environment Withdrawing the emotional energy of the relationship to re-invest it elsewhere

However, *Figure 23.1.1* is also a simple model, and in practice grief does not move in straight lines. A more dynamic model describes the bereaved individual oscillating between two processes: the activities and pain of letting go; and the adaptation and change of the restoration–orientated process (*Figure 23.1.2*).

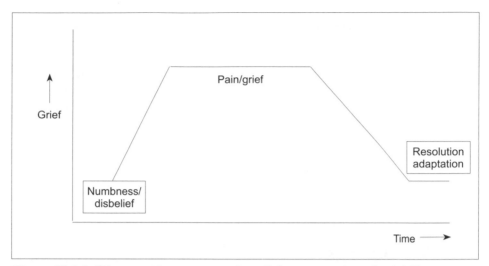

Figure 23.1.1: Diagramatic representation of the progression of grief. From Faulkner and Maguire (1994)

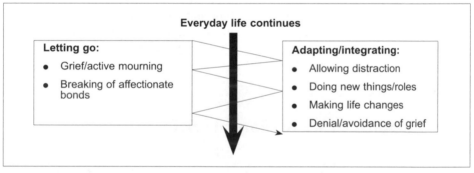

Figure 23.1.2 The two processes of bereavement. From Stroebe and Schut (1995)

The depth and duration of the grief vary greatly, depending on:

- the closeness of the relationship
- the type of death
- the personality of the bereaved
- expectations of society
- spiritual or religious belief.

23.2 Anticipatory grief

Grieving can start as soon as the reality of the loss is accepted. In palliative care settings, this may happen any time from diagnosis onwards and it is not uncommon for both patient and family to grieve together. Sometimes, especially after a prolonged illness, much of the grieving has been done by the time the patient dies, and the survivor may be surprised to find the overwhelming emotion is one of relief rather than grief. This needs to be differentiated from absent grief, where there is no grief reaction at any stage.

23.3 Anniversaries

It is almost universal that there may be a resurgence of acute grief around the time of the anniversary of the death. The first anniversary can be particularly difficult, and the bereaved person often finds themselves re-visiting the events of the year before with their attendant emotions in a painful way. Sometimes this can persist, to a lesser degree, for many years. It is common to recognize the anniversary of a death in some way, and this may aid the grieving process.

23.4 Supportive care for normal grief

There is no evidence of any sort of structured intervention that affects the outcome of 'normal' grief. However, the bereaved both appreciate and expect contact (telephone, visit or letter) from the primary healthcare team, especially the GP. If this is not given, it can be perceived as abandonment and cause great distress. A letter of sympathy or a simple acknowledgement of the loss is often all that is required, although there may also be a need for additional information. Most doctors recognize this need.

A bereavement consultation might contain:

- an expression of sympathy
- offer of help — 'Is there anything practical I can do to help?' With an offer to follow up if required
- an offer to discuss the cause of death and any outstanding questions
- identification of those at risk of variant grief reactions

- the provision of more structured support for those at risk of variant grief reactions
- some written guidance on the grieving process and any local support services
- encourage expression of emotion
- leaving the door open.

This consultation is usually remembered with gratitude for many years, although it is not always easy for the GP.

There may be a question about the prescribing of benzodiazepines or night sedatives in the early days. Generally this is to be discouraged; it can suppress emotional expression and the normal grieving process. Occasionally a small amount of night sedation can help if there is major sleep disturbance.

Some practices set up systems to identify the bereaved and tag the case notes in some way, or record a recent death on the problem list or summary page. This is particularly useful in large, multi-doctor practices, so the bereaved person does not constantly have to explain his or her predicament.

Modern British culture has been described as 'death denying', and it is common for the bereaved to describe intense social isolation and a sense that even those closest to them do not know what to say; they either avoid the subject or, still more painfully, avoid the bereaved person.

> *The grief was so acute that if people came in and didn't talk about him, in order not to upset me, it upset me that they didn't mention him.*

> Bereaved woman

Bereavement support groups exist in most areas. They offer volunteer befriending and counselling services, and volunteers are usually offered a good level of training and supervision. Many hospices offer bereavement services, as do churches, some social services departments and voluntary agencies such as Cruse, SANDS (for stillbirths, miscarriages and neonatal deaths) and the Compassionate Friends (for the death of a child). The practice counsellor or a local counselling service may feel able to offer bereavement support.

There is much debate about what constitutes 'normal' behaviour after a bereavement, and to what extent a universal human experience should be medicalized. However, a few people do develop significant problems relating to loss and bereavement that may benefit from skilled therapeutic intervention.

23.5 Abnormal grief (*Table 23.5.1*)

Table 23.5.1: Abnormal grief			
Name of variant	Clinical picture	'Stage' where grief is struck	Possible other explanations
Absent grief	The bereaved person carries on with no observable grief	Unconscious denial or active blocking of emotional response (stage 1–2, transition)	Anticipatory grief completed Hidden grief (grieving in secret) Insignificant relationship (eg. empty marriage)
Delayed grief	The bereaved person appears to carry on as usual, then something 'triggers' an emotional reaction	Conscious denial or active blocking of emotional response (stage 1–2, transition)	Hidden grief (grieving in secret) Excessive stoicism Overburdened with responsibility (eg. single parent, main income source)
Chronic grief	The grief appears to continue unabated	No adaptation/resolution (stage 2–3, transition)	Different cultural norms Emotional/dramatic personality

23.6 Identifying those at risk of abnormal grief

Risk factors have been described for variant grief reactions (delayed or absent grief and chronic grief). They are:

- very dependent relationships
- relationships with a lot of mixed feelings/ambivalence ('stormy' relationships)
- sudden or violent death
- untimely death — the loss of a child, adolescent or young adult
- suicide
- feeling unsupported
- other major problems, such as economic worries
- pre-existing or previous significant mental health problems
- multiple bereavements.

Those at risk should be followed up. Some argue that all bereaved people should be followed up six weeks after the death to allow better assessment. Where abnormal grief or clinical depression is present, referral to a clinical psychology or psychiatric service may be appropriate.

23.7 Addressing the primary care team bereavement needs

Primary care team members may also grieve the death of a patient, particularly if the relationship goes back many years or involvement has been intense. Almost all GPs in one study also described feelings of guilt or self-blame related to fears of making or having made mistakes in the general practice environment. Many also describe grief at the death of patients they may have known over many years. This should be acknowledged and supported.

23.8 Bereavement and children (see also section *14.7* on families)

Children and teenagers also experience bereavement. Sometimes their needs are less well acknowledged or met because:

- of a belief that children do not experience grief
- of a desire to spare them pain
- there is often simultaneous bereavement of their parent(s).

Children start to form a concept of death from age two to three years onwards. This gradually matures and is often fully formed by the age of about eight years.

Children grieve. Sometimes the natural protective instinct of the surviving parent is to disguise what has happened in some way to lessen its impact on the child, or even to send the child away to 'spare them' the distress. This tends to produce confusion, fear, anger and psychological sequelae.

Generally, children benefit from:

⌘ Being involved in what is happening, with simple, truthful explanations they can understand (avoiding euphemisms such as 'daddy's gone to sleep, he's not coming back', which can leave a deep fear of sleep, as well as incomprehension).
⌘ Being given opportunity to be involved in rituals around death, choosing flowers or wreaths, writing personal messages, being a part of the funeral.
⌘ Being allowed and encouraged to express emotion. Seeing a surviving parent cry can help this ('I am crying because I am sad and miss daddy very much'), yet the parent will often struggle to maintain a brave face.

⌘ Being allowed and encouraged to talk about the dead person. Making photograph albums, memory books or being given a special possession or item of clothing that belonged to the dead person can help.

⌘ Maintaining the familiar regimen. Ritual and habit comfort the whole family. Children and teenagers do not always grieve in the sustained way adults do — they may get engrossed in play, in school work, in social activity. This does not mean they have forgotten or that they are quickly over it.

⌘ Being allowed to regress in their behaviour and needs for a while.

The surviving parent is the key supporter of his or her child, and it is important to work through the parent and support him or her. Encourage networks in the family, friends, neighbours, a teacher at school, who can all give the child additional support.

Additional support may be available from the health visitor, social services, some palliative care services and child psychology services.

Key points

❖ Bereavement, the loss of someone dearly loved, is one the most painful human experiences.

❖ Grief is associated with increased rates of both physical and mental illness, and increased mortality.

❖ Grief may vary in time course and in intensity and depth.

❖ Grieving can start as soon as the reality of the loss is accepted. This is sometimes before the death.

❖ There is commonly a resurgence of acute grief around the time of the anniversary of the death.

❖ The newly bereaved both appreciate and expect contact from the primary healthcare team, especially the GP.

❖ Normal grief often needs no intervention, apart from supportive care.

❖ Abnormal grief needs skilled therapeutic intervention.

❖ Children and teenagers also grieve, but their needs may be less well met.

Reference

Faulkner A, Maguire P (1994) *Talking to Cancer Patients and their Relatives*. Oxford Medical Publications, Oxford

Further reading

Charlton R, Dolman E (1995) Bereavement: a protocol for primary care. *Br J Gen Pract* **45**: 427–30

Main J (2000) Improving management of bereavement in general practice based on a survey of recently bereaved subjects in a single general practice. *Br J Gen Pract* **50**: 863–6

Rees D (1997) *Death and Bereavement*. Whurr publishers, London

Ringdal G, Ringdal K, Kaasda S (2001) The first year of grief and bereavement in close family members to individuals who have died of cancer. *Palliat Med* **15**: 91–105

Saunderson EM, Ridsdale L (1999) General practitioners beliefs and attitudes about how to respond to death and bereavement: qualitative study. *Br Med J* **319**: 293–6

Sheldon F (1998) ABC of palliative care: bereavement. *Br Med J* **316**: 456–8

Stroebe M, Stroebe W, Hansson R, Schut H (2001) *Handbook of Bereavement Research: consequences, coping and care*. American Psychological Association, Washington

Twycross R (1995) *Introducing Palliative Care*. Radcliffe Medical Press, Oxford

Worden W (1991) *Grief and Grief Counselling*. Routledge, London

Part 5
Organisational aspects

24

The general practice and primary care team

24.1 A practice checklist

⌘ Do you hold regular, multidisciplinary, clinical team meetings?

⌘ Do you identify patients requiring palliative care during these meetings?

⌘ Does your practice 'design in' good communication and mutual support?

⌘ Have you established rapid access for these patients, such as a computer alert saying 'rapid access' (to prompt receptionists to fit them in)?

⌘ Have you effective systems for handover when someone is off or on holiday?

⌘ Have you someone in the practice team with an interest in palliative care who can be a resource for others?

⌘ Have you got rapid access to syringe drivers and syringe driver drugs during normal hours?

⌘ Have you got proper stock control and documentation of controlled drugs in your practice?

⌘ Have you rapid access to equipment such as commodes and beds?

⌘ Do you leave written information with patients about how to access in-hours and out-of-hours services?

⌘ Do you leave written information for patients about what medication they can administer and when?

⌘ Do you leave written information about benefits?

⌘ Do the family know how to handle the patient, such as turning?

⌘ Do you anticipate problems or simply react to them as they arise?

⌘ Do you carry a resource pack (information about syringe driver drug doses, telephone numbers of specialist services, etc.) in your bag?

⌘ Do you have a handover form to notify the out-of-hours services?

⌘ Do you routinely write a bereavement letter to bereaved families?

⌘ Do you give written information about local bereavement services?

⌘ Do you hold a team de-brief on difficult or traumatic cases?

⌘ Do you support each other with regular, informal de-briefing?

24.2 Identifying palliative care patients

Most practices will identify and review patients requiring palliative care at the practice clinical team meeting. Identifying such patients from the practice computer for audit purposes is less straightforward.

Computer searches only reflect the data entered in the first place. Most practices do not use the codes for palliative care, and patients are coded under the original diagnosis, such as carcinoma of the bronchus. Palliative care describes a phase in the patient journey rather than a diagnosis.

The new GMS GP contract has quality payments available for identifying cancer payments. Use this list of patients and a list of non-cancer diagnoses, such as heart failure, as a starting point to identify those needing palliative care. Go looking for these patients, rather than waiting for them to present.

24.3 Working as a team

Effective team working

Effective team working is critically important in palliative care. A dysfunctional team with poor communication will compromise the care delivered. One of the problems is that we are all so busy. The busier and more pressured it becomes, the more important leadership becomes. Someone needs to step back and take an overview. Is the way the primary care team is working, communicating and using its scarce resources likely to be effective in palliative care? Is everyone under so much pressure that the non-medical aspects of care, such as listening and kindness, get lost?

One of the most effective initiatives could be to reorganize the delivery of in-hours care for minor illness and free up the clinicians for more complex issues such as palliative care. We need to 'design in' some spare capacity, as palliative care creates a sudden significant increase in demand on our time and we frequently only get one chance to get it right.

Communication and confidentiality

There may be a tension between good communication and confidentiality, especially if the 'team' includes lay members such as spiritual leaders or voluntary agencies. It is good practice to get (and document) the patient's consent for discussion outside the clinical team. This is discussed in more detail in *Chapter 16.5*.

Rapid access

The non-clinical team in the practice need to be able to recognise patients who need rapid access. A patient on chemotherapy with a sore throat and fever should not be offered an appointment for the following week. The non-clinical team do not need to know the clinical details, simply whether that patient should be seen that day. A simple alert on the computer saying 'rapid access' helps.

Practice culture

The primary care team consists of people. It is less effective if half the workforce is off sick with stress. We all have our strengths and weaknesses, and we bring personal beliefs and experience to every palliative care situation. Death raises many questions and uncertainties, and certain situations may prove distressing for members of the team and get underneath the professional 'protective shield'. The professionals involved should 'look out' for each other. This may be stating the obvious, but it is often not done effectively. The practice needs to 'design in' the mutual support as much as possible. Part-time workers in particular can become isolated from the team. Formal and structured meetings and de-briefings are useful, but the fact that a team always meets for coffee at 11.30 every morning may be equally effective. This mutual support needs to be part of the practice culture.

Links with the wider team

The primary care team acts as a gateway to other services. Good links with the specialist palliative care services, the community palliative care services, occupational therapists and physiotherapists are essential. Whenever a palliative care patient is reviewed, a standard question should be 'Is it time to involve more specialist services?'. It is usually better to involve the specialist services earlier rather than later. Palliative care is very much about keeping one step ahead and anticipating the next move.

Understanding roles

Good team working is enhanced by good understanding of each other's roles, strengths and limitations. This needs clear communication with each other, but can then avoid both wasteful duplication and the frustration of unreasonable expectation. It is important to clarify who the key worker is for the patient, who can take an overview and coordinate other primary care, secondary care and specialist palliative care input. This is usually the GP, but may be the district nurse, the specialist palliative care nurse or others.

24.4 Significant event audit in palliative care

Many practices already have adverse incident reporting (AIR), a system of reporting problems or near misses. This is reactive and is triggered by something going wrong.

Significant event audit (SEA) is different. It is the analysis of an event proactively to see what can be learnt from the way it was handled. It may well highlight examples of excellent care (we can learn from when it goes well as well as from our mistakes). Should we go by 'SEA' or 'AIR'? The simple answer is both.

An episode of palliative care lends itself well to significant event audit. The process can be team building and it can identify 'system' weaknesses. Simple audit can also be useful — in what place are your patients dying?

Key points
- Use the checklist above to check how you manage palliative care.
- Functional teams provide better care and better communication.
- Ensure 'rapid access' for palliative care patients.
- Implement significant event audit for palliative care.

25

Out-of-hours palliative care

Two-thirds of every week is classed as 'out of hours' (OOH). The OOH period spans 105.5 hours per week, between 18.30 every weekday evening to 08.00 the following morning, and from 18.30 Friday evening to 08.00 on Monday morning. In-hours care spans just 52.5 hours.

Over the past twenty years we have seen a transition from most GPs delivering personal care twenty-four hours-a-day, to organizations covering large groups of GPs. It is likely today that the doctor called to see the terminally ill patient in the OOH period will be a stranger and will not have access to his or her clinical record. The continuity of care for a terminally ill patient is, therefore, easily broken in the OOH period. There may be ten or more shifts of doctors during a weekend; fourteen on a bank holiday.

The whole structure of OOH primary care has changed further with the new GP contract. Many GPs will opt out of OOH working. These GP OOH cooperatives and commercial OOH providers of care will have to evolve to become 'community OOH service providers'. These new organizations are likely to have a different skill mix (less doctors, more nurses and other health professionals).

There is an opportunity here for OOH services to no longer be viewed as a series of vertical hierarchies (eg. GPs, district nursing services, social services, mental health teams), rather as a fully-integrated OOH team (*Figure 25.1*). The primary care organizations (primary care trusts [PCTs] in England) can commission it as such.

Where does palliative care fit into this? The danger is that the care could become even more fragmented. It is essential that:

※ There is effective identification of a patient needing palliative care. This could be done by making them 'special patients' highlighted on the OOH database. This requires effective communication of such patients to the OOH provider.
※ An effective system of handover of such patients from in-hours services to OOH services and back again is developed.
※ The palliative care training needs for those working OOH are met
※ The OOH provider is properly equipped to deal with palliative care patients at home.

⌘ The OOH service is designed to help palliative care patients to stay at home when they wish. This requires the appropriate skill mix and may involve the inclusion of palliative care nurses in the OOH team

⌘ Pro-active care in-hours is strengthened to avoid crises during the OOH period.

See *Figure 25.2* for an example of an OOH handover form.

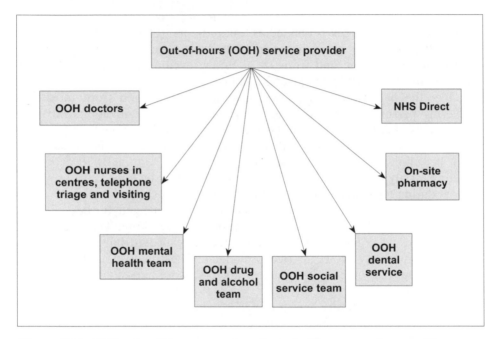

Figure 25.1: Skill mix of the new community out-of-hours service providers

Palliative care handover form and night nursing service referral

Information from GP/District Nurse/Macmillan Nurse to out-of-hours services about patients with palliative care needs.

Please fax/send to Cuedoc (01228 402803) **and** leave a copy with the patient

PATIENT DETAILS

Date ....

Name of patient .... DOB ....
Address ....
....
Main carer ....
....
....

Night nursing service

Home visit required: ☐
Approximate time: ....
Reason for visit: ....
....
Directions: ....
....
Person making referral:
....

MEDICAL/NURSING DETAILS

Diagnosis .... GP ....
Complicating conditions ....
Known wishes of patient and family, eg. re place of care, further treatments, etc
....
Current hospital treatment, eg. chemo/radiotherapy ....
Services involved: Palliative care consultant ....
                   Macmillan nurse: .... District Nurse: ....
                   Other consultants: .... Hospice: ....

PROGRESS

eg. regular and PRN medication, changes to medication, patient's insight, plans for weekend, plans for anticipated problems

Date		Signed

Figure 25.2: Out-of-hours handover form

There can be significant problems accessing palliative care drugs quickly OOH. A relatively small and predictable range of drugs will allow most symptoms to be addressed at home. This avoids the sort of situation described below.

> *By Sunday morning he was in much pain. He was having great difficulty actually getting the number of tablets down. The nurse arranged a prescription. My daughters had to drive a round trip of fifty miles to collect the prescription, then the drugs for the district nurse to set up the syringe driver. This was very upsetting for them as they wanted to stay with him. The dexamethasone injection was not available and they were asked to go back the next day. He was made comfortable. Three hours later he was in severe pain. The person who answered the phone number the nurse had given us said, 'It's Sunday and the pharmacies are closed.'*
>
> *We gave a subcutaneous injection of diamorphine ourselves. He was still in severe pain when, about fifteen minutes later, he died in our arms.*
>
> *I feel terrible about all this as I feel it is partly my profession that has allowed these terrible situations to happen. Please can we try to prevent it happening again, particularly to a young person. He was such a lovely boy.*
>
> Mother of a nineteen-year-old boy who died
> of metastatic melanoma on a Sunday

The commonest drugs needed OOH are:

- diamorphine 10 mg, 30 mg and 100 mg injection (see 'Accessing controlled drugs OOH' below)
- cyclizine 50 mg injection
- haloperidol 5 mg injection
- metoclopramide 10 mg injection
- levomepromazine (Nozinan®) 25 mg injection
- midazolam 10 mg injection
- hyoscine hydrobromide 400 µg injection (or glycopyrrollate 0.4 mg/2 ml injection)
- water for injections.

Less commonly used are:

- dexamethasone 20 mg/5 ml injection
- diazepam 10 mg rectally or 10 mg/2 ml injection intravenously
- ketorolac 30 mg/ml injection
- oxygen.

A Department of Health implementation group is working on OOH rapid access to palliative care drugs, and guidance should be available soon. Ways to improve access include:

⌘ Prescribing an 'emergency pack' on a named-patient basis, which is left in the patient's home. This allows controlled drugs to be included. The handover form can contain a reminder.
⌘ PCTs or OOH services recruiting/paying a team of community pharmacists to carry an identified range of palliative care drugs and provide a rapid access on-call rota. Again this allows access to controlled drugs.
⌘ Using nominated pharmacies, community hospitals, acute hospitals, hospices or the OOH service base to carry palliative care emergency drug packs (excludes controlled drugs).
⌘ Carrying a 'palliative care kit' in the OOH service car (see *Figure 25.3*). A kit can also carry equipment such as syringe drivers, syringes, catheterization packs and local symptom management guidelines (excludes controlled drugs).

I didn't know there was a palliative care box in the GP co-operative cars.

GP (2001) at a teaching session on OOH palliative care

Whatever option is used, a key to success is that all OOH team members are fully aware of how the medication is accessed in the locality in which they are working. A well-equipped palliative care kit in the boot of the car or a local pharmacy will only make a difference if it is accessed and used when needed.

⌘ Graseby syringe driver kit with giving set and spare batteries.

⌘ Information sheets on doses for syringe drivers and instructions on use of syringe driver.

⌘ Midazolam injection.

⌘ Hysocine hydrobromide injection.

⌘ Ketorolac injection.

⌘ Haloperidol injection.

⌘ Metoclopramide injection.

⌘ Cyclizine injection.

⌘ Levomepromazine injection.

⌘ Water for injection 10 ml.

Figure 25.3: An OOH palliative care kit, which should be carried in each car. From CueDoc — The North Cumbria Cooperative

Accessing controlled drugs OOH

The OOH provider needs to have clear guidance on how to access controlled drugs OOH. If the provider chooses to carry such drugs themselves, they must find a solution to the prospect of perhaps 200 doctors having access. In addition, they would have to apply for a home office licence to buy and dispense such drugs. Unless legislation changes, it is more practical for individual doctors to carry their own opioid in their doctor's bag (for example, five vials of diamorphine 10 mg). This is, of course, also necessary for cardiac chest pain and other severe pains. It would be sufficient for most starting doses of a syringe driver.

The alternatives are:

• to prescribe drugs pro-actively on a named-patient basis and leave them in the house
• to use local community hospitals as a resource
• to use local general hospitals (eg. accident and emergency departments) as a resource
• to have arrangements with the local pharmacists
• to use local hospices.

Documentation needs to be meticulous.

The role of NHS Direct in OOH service provision

Another 'player' has been introduced into the already complex system of OOH service provision. It is the Government's stated aim that all calls from patients OOH will be routed via NHS Direct. The call handler may be 100 miles away, and the nurse may be sitting in a control room at the other end of the country with no knowledge of the local services. NHS Direct nurses use a decision support software system that is risk averse. The problem with this is '999 ambulances' can be triggered and accident and emergency attendance arranged inappropriately when these algorithms are applied to palliative care. There is a strong case for palliative care patients to be routed straight to the local OOH service provider, rather than having NHS Direct nurse triage.

Supporting carers in the OOH period

By providing adequate support to carers and relatives we can often avoid care breakdown and admission. Access to support should be made as easy as possible for carers. It's not just the elderly and frail that find the prospect of accessing OOH services daunting. Some GPs and nurses still give patients their home telephone numbers for the OOH period to ensure continuity; if a patient is known to one of the voluntary services then contact numbers are often left. Despite this, lack of support to carers has been identified as one of the key causes of uneccessary admission. How can we solve this?

The new multidisciplinary OOH service providers offer an opportunity. There needs to be a clear strategy within that organisation to manage palliative care patients. In many areas there is still no access to twenty-four-hour general nursing cover, never mind specialist palliative care nursing teams. The new OOH general nursing team could, however, be organized to have at least one nurse with palliative care training. This nurse could carry a mobile telephone, the direct line number of which could be given to patients and carers. This would avoid the multi-step process of accessing the OOH system, and the nurse will have good knowledge of local resources. This number could be given to patients and their carers as part of the written information about how to access care. Local hospices could provide an alternative source of OOH advice to patients and their carers.

Local availability of and access to crisis response teams, Hospice-at-Home nursing services, Marie Curie nurses and larger items of equipment OOH needs to be clear. As with OOH drugs, the information needs to be easily available to the OOH doctor or nurse in the middle of the night.

Resources for the practice

Books

General symptom control/overview

Twycross R (2002) *Introducing Palliative Care*. 4th edn. Radcliffe Medical Press, Oxford

Regnard C (2002) *Supportive and Palliative Care in Cancer: An introduction*. Radcliffe Medical Press, Oxford

Lugton J, Kindlen M, eds (1999) *Palliative care. The Nursing Role*. Churchill Livingstone, Edinburgh

Twycross R, Wilcock (2001) *Symptom Management in Advanced Cancer*. 3rd edn. Radcliffe Medical Press, Oxford

Regnard C, Hockley J (2003) *A Guide to Symptom Relief in Palliative Care*. 5th edn. Radcliffe Medical Press, Oxford

Fallon M, O'Neill B, eds (1988) *ABC of Palliative Care*. BMJ Books, London

Kaye P (1994) *A–Z Pocketbook of Symptom Control*. EPL Publications, Northampton

Palliative care in primary care

Faull C, Carter Y, Daniels L, eds (2005) *The Handbook of Palliative Care*. Blackwell Science (UK), Oxford

Charlton R, ed (2002) *Primary Palliative Care*. Radcliffe Medical Press, Oxford

Doyle D (1994) *Domiciliary Palliative care: A handbook for family doctors and community nurses* (Oxford General Practice No 27). Oxford University Press, Oxford

Prescribing

Twycross R, Wilcock A , Thorp S (2002) *Palliative Care Formulary*. 2nd edn. Radcliffe Medical Press, Oxford

Dying

Ellershaw J, Wilkinson S (2003) *Care for the Dying: A pathway to excellence*. Oxford University Press, Oxford

Thomas K (2003) *Caring for the Dying at Home*. Radcliffe Medical Press, Oxford

For families

Doyle D (1994) *Caring for a Dying Relative*. Oxford University Press, Oxford

Lynn J, Harris J (1999) *Handbook for Mortals: Guidance for people facing serious illness*. Oxford University Press, Oxford

Useful websites

For printer friendly downloads of selected charts from this book: North Cumbria Palliative care services website: www.northcumbriahealth.nhs.uk/palliativecare

For more information about palliative care services with addresses and useful links: Hospice Information Service: www.hospiceinformation.info

National Council for hospice and specialist palliative care services: www.hospice-spc-council.org.uk/

Palliative medicine matters. Book catalogue, links, syringe driver prescribing information: www.pallmed.net/index

National Forum for Hospice at Home: www.HospiceAtHome.org.uk

Macmillan Cancer Relief: www.macmillan.org.uk

Marie Curie Cancer Care: www.mariecurie.org.uk

Scottish Partnership for Palliative Care: www.palliativecarescotland.org.uk

International Association for Hospice and Palliative Care (includes on-line palliative care manual): www.hospicecare.com

For more information about symptom control:

British Medical Journal collected resources on Palliative Medicine: www./bmj.com/cgi/collection/palliative_medicine

'ABC of palliative care' BMJ book on-line: www.hospice-spc-council.org.uk/informat.ion/abcofpc

Palliative care links and resource material (Canadian site linking to multiple high quality palliative care resources and guidelines): www.palliative.info

Education for physicians on end-of-life care. Major US project, including downloadable training manual: www.epec.net

For more information about cancer:

BACUP (British Association of Cancer United Patients): www.cancerbacup.org.uk

University of Newcastle UK guide to internet resources for cancer: www.cancerindex.org

National Cancer Institute (major US review articles): www.cancer.gov/cancer_information

For more information about non-cancer diagnoses:

Alzheimers society: www.alzheimers.org.uk

Motor Neurone disease Association: www.mndassociation.org

Multiple Sclerosis Society: www.mssociety.org.uk

Parkinsons disease society: www.parkinsons.org.uk

Stroke association: www.stroke.org.uk

Terrence Higgins Trust (AIDS or HIV infection): www.tht.org.uk

British Heart Foundation: www.bhf.org.uk

For more information about prescribing and therapeutics:

Palliative care formulary. Includes syringe driver drug compatibility charts: www.palliativedrugs.com

Palliative medicine matters. Book catalogue, links, syringe driver prescribing information: www.pallmed.net/index

For more information about complementary therapies:

British Medical Journal collected resources on complementary therapies: www.bmj.com/cgi/collection/complementary_medicine

National Cancer Institute (Major US review articles): www.cancer.gov/cancer_information/list.aspx?

Foundation for integrated medicine (links to Department of Health guidelines on complementary therapies in Primary Care): www.fimed.org

For more information about religion/spirituality:

Hospital chaplaincy site providing links to many religious/spiritual sites: www.hospitalchaplain.com

Virtual religions index. Major academic site covering all religions: www.religion.rutgers.edu/vri/index.html

Non-academic interfaith site: www.beliefnet.com

For more information about death and dying:

Death:an enquiry into mans mortal weakness: www.library.advanced.org/16665/cgi-bin/index.cgi

Death and dying: www.dying.about.com

Natural death centre, 'aims to support those dying at home and their carers and to help people to arrange inexpensive, do-it-yourself and environmentally-friendly funerals. It

has a more general aim of helping to improve the quality of dying.'
www.naturaldeath.org.uk

For more information about grief/bereavement:

Crisis, grief and healing: www.webhealing.com

Cruse bereavement care: www.crusebereavement.org.uk

London Bereavement Network: www.bereavement.org.uk

Childhood bereavement network. Access from and search for services in your locality: www.ncb.org.uk

Compassionate friends (for bereaved parents): www.tcf.org.uk

The Child death helpline (Great Ormond Street Hospital): www.childdeathhelpline.org

Specialist palliative care services

All these services are developing rapidly across the UK. Many are voluntary and develop in response to locally perceived need, but increasingly, joint NHS/voluntary sector partnerships are providing more closely integrated services.

Not all services are available in all areas, but most are willing to give telephone advice. The Hospice Information Service (St Christophers Hospice, Tel 0870 903 3903 or www.hospiceinformation.info) collates an up to date database of services across the UK and Ireland.

Sometimes there is confusion, particularly between different parts of the nursing services over who does what. Some specialist community nursing services offer advice/ support, some can offer hands-on care for longer periods of time.

In-patient hospices/palliative care units

Offer inpatient care for patients with advanced, life-threatening illness. May be NHS or voluntary, but usually staffed by doctors, nurses and other professionals with skill and expertise in physical, psychological, social and spiritual care. Many offer other services such as day care, lymphoedema services, outpatient clinics, home care, complementary therapies, bereavement services.

Day hospices

These may be attached to an in-patient unit, or freestanding. Allow palliative care assessment and input for patients wanting to stay at home, while offering carer respite.
Services vary, but may include:

- medical and nursing care and advice
- recreational, creative and complementary therapies
- active rehabilitation with physiotherapy and occupational therapy input
- social activities
- carer education/support.

Hospice at Home services — hands-on role

These teams aim to provide nursing, and sometimes specialised medical care, in the patient's home. They provide sufficient, additional hands-on nursing care to allow patients, who would otherwise have needed admission, to stay in their own home. This may be for a crisis, pain and symptom control, respite or care during dying, depending on local referral criteria. Availability, staffing levels and skill mix vary. Many also offer loan equipment, and work closely with the primary healthcare teams, and community specialist nurses.

Specialist palliative care home care nurses (Macmillan nurses) — advisory role

They provide expertise in pain/symptom control, emotional and family support, both directly to patients and their families and also, increasingly, by educating and supporting the primary care team. They offer a good link with other parts of the specialist services. They are usually available 9–5pm, Monday to Friday, occasionally twenty-four-hour rota.

Marie Curie nurses — hands-on role

These nurses are organised and, partly funded, by the Marie Curie Cancer Care to provide one-to-one hands-on nursing care for shifts in the patient's home. The service is usually for patients with cancer. Availability varies, care is usually arranged through the district nurses.

Hospital support teams — advisory role

Specialist nurses, increasingly supported by specialist doctors, social workers or other staff provide help and advice, expertise in pain/symptom control, emotional and family support, both directly to patients and their families and to the hospital teams caring for them. Discharge planning is usually seen as important, so team members will often ask to speak with the GP and district nursing staff prior to complex discharges.

Palliative care outpatient clinics

Held in hospitals, hospices or community hospitals. Usually referral is doctor-to-doctor, from the GP or hospital consultant to the palliative care consultant. A palliative care assessment will include advice on interventions to maximise physical comfort, emotional adjustment and family issues. A specialist nurse may also be involved in the assessment.

Increasingly, nurse-led clinics may address specific areas, such as breathlessness, or lymphoedema.

Pain services may also offer outpatient assessment for interventional anaesthesia.

Lymphoedema services

These are nurse-led, physiotherapy-led or multidisciplinary outpatient clinics. Access varies across the UK.

The lymphoedema support network (www.lymphoedema.org) carries global links, the British lymphology society (www.lymphoedema.org/bls/) carries an up-to-date directory of UK services and the referral pathways.

Bereavement services

These may be linked to other specialist providers, such as hospices or Macmillan teams, social services or voluntary agencies, for example, Cruse.

Services vary widely. There may be telephone contact, bereavement visiting, a bereavement group, one-to-one or family counselling, access to complementary therapies, and links with other agencies. Some hospices or children's services have developed specific services for bereaved children.

A brief palliative care consultation checklist

Physical:

- ❖ Pain?
- ❖ Breathlessness, cough?
- ❖ Constipation?
- ❖ Continence?
- ❖ Itch?
- ❖ Mouth problems?
- ❖ Anorexia and nutrition?
- ❖ Fatigue?
- ❖ Medication review needed?

Psychological:

- ❖ Fear?
- ❖ Anxiety?
- ❖ Depression?
- ❖ Insomnia?

Social:

- ❖ Effect on family?
- ❖ Benefits And other social support needs?
- ❖ Sexuality?

Spritual:

- ❖ What does this mean for them?

Organizational:

- ❖ Follow up?
- ❖ Safety netting?
- ❖ Anticipating next step?
- ❖ Access in hours and out of hours?
- ❖ Communication within the team?

Index

micro-enema 55, 56
midazolam 44, 53, 55, 56, ,
61, 64, 88, 177
minority groups 218, 219,
220, 221, 223, 224
mobility
loss of 101
mood disorders 162
morale 89, 112
moral principles 200
Morcap 16
morphgesic 16
morphine 57, 52, 103, 63,
102, 104, 52, 53, 57,
12, 51
common fears and concerns
13
myths 14
patient information leaflet 22
prescribing 15
prescribing checklist 21
rapid dose escalation 18
severe pain 18
side-effects 27, 36
topical 63
morphine formulations 16
immediate-release, modi-
fied-release 15
morphine oral solution 16
motor neurone disease
(MND) 98, 100, 104,
105, 111
mourning 154, 162, 266,
268, 269
rituals 266
mouthwashes 77
mouth care 209
mouth ulcers 77
MST 16
mucolytics 57
multidisciplinary team 62
multifocal myoclonus 104
multiple sclerosis 100, 104
multiprofessional team 114,
120

multisystem disease 100
muscle spasm 37, 40, , 104
muscle weakness 66
muscular dystrophies 219
mutilation 224
MXL 16
myeloma 66

N

nasogastric tube 50, 82
nausea 83, 82, 80, 79, 65, 59,
101, 194, 49,
causes 79
nausea and vomiting
morphine induced 17
syringe driver 81
nebulized saline 65
nerve blocks 115
coelic or splanchnic 41
intercostal 41
nerve compression pain 37
nerve destruction pain 37
nerve pain 9, 10, 11, 24,
35, 39
neurodegenerative disorders
219
neurological disease 104,
111
neuropathic pain 109
neuropathies 109
NHS walk-in centres 224
nifedipine 65
nightmares 172
nocturia 172
non-cancer diagnoses 116
non-cancer palliative care
general principles 98
non-drug interventions 18,
35, 41
non-steroidal anti-inflammatory drugs 34, 37,
87, 134
non-treatment decisions 205
non-verbal clues 159

nourishment 89
numbness 82, 155
nurse specialists 98
nursing care 122
nursing homes 117
nurturing 89
nutrition 89
as death approaches 96
prevention of cancer 89
nutritional supplements 91
nutritional support
for the patient with reduced
appetite 92
nystatin 78

O

'out-of-hours' teams 126
occupational therapists 41,
60, 203
octreotide , 50, 58, 82, 83
odour , 62, 63, 69
odour-absorbent dressings 62
oedema 72, 74, 75, , 76
causes of 72
openness 98
opioids 5, 9, 10, 11, 12, 13,
14, 18, 20, 25, 26, 27,
28, 29, 30, 31, 32, 33,
34, 35, 36, 38, 41, 42,
43, 45, 172, 176
opioid analgesics 134
opioid rotation 27, 35
oramorph 16, 22, 26, 30,
31, 42
out-of-hours palliative care
283
out-of-hours service 28
out-of-hours services 115
ovarian cancer 48
oxybutinin 70
oxycodone 28, 31, 35, 36
oxycodone injection 29